What people are

Zero Waste Living

When most of us ponder what we can do about climate change and pollution, we fall into a dark pit of personal guilt and helplessness. Stephanie Miller reaches a helping hand right into the pit and pulls us up with her practical ideas and can-do attitude. She shows us by example, in frank and friendly prose, how to get a grip on our personal waste stream—eating, composting, reusing and recycling in creative ways to save ourselves and the planet.

Melanie Choukas-Bradley, author of *Finding Solace at Theodore Roosevelt Island* and *Resilience: Connecting with Nature in a Time of Crisis*

Stephanie Miller has illuminated a global human imperative – waste can no longer be tolerated. Her practical guidance shows how we can institutionalize waste reduction in our homes. It also exposes the environmental impacts of our food system – and how wasting food is one of the most environmentally detrimental habits we can no longer ignore.

Pete Pearson, Senior Director for Food Waste, World Wildlife Fund

I knew our planet and its people couldn't handle much more wasteful consumption. Until reading Stephanie Miller's book, I didn't know what to do—I felt too busy and flawed to take up the fight against waste. This book gives practical and easy ideas that helped me overcome my fatalism. Reading it, I felt I could live better and be part of something bigger, perhaps catch up with a better future. Looking forward to seeing you there.

Paul O'Brien, Vice President, Policy and Advocacy, Oxfam America and author of *Power Switch*

Stephanie helps us see what we can do every day to make a significant difference to our environment. Her 80/20 approach is very refreshing and easy to follow. She offers universally simple but powerful solutions. This book should have a central place in each household that wants to make a difference and help us save our planet for new generations.

Nena Stoiljkovic, Regional Vice President for Asia and Pacific, International Finance Corporation

Stephanie Miller gives us an insightful and practical approach on how to meaningfully play our role in the climate change fight. Based on her extensive and successful professional experience as a climate change champion, she knows how to relate to the choices that we make every day whether when buying groceries or managing our usage of plastics. This page-turner makes us pause and rethink most of our daily gestures.

Sérgio Pimenta, Regional Vice President for Middle East and Africa, International Finance Corporation

Congrats to Stephanie on writing an engaging, fun, and pragmatic guide to zero waste living! There are ideas and strategies here that any household can adopt. It's a delightful and informative read.

Catherine Plume, Zero Waste advocate and Chair, D.C. Chapter of Sierra Club

Stephanie was a leading voice on climate change mitigation at the World Bank Group, and it's wonderful to see how she has used her expertise and experience to create this very practical guide on how each individual, even with daily tight schedules, may have a positive impact on the environment.

Anne N. Kabagambe, Executive Director at the World Bank Group and author of *A Global Playbook for the Next Pandemic*

Stephanie provides readers with a wonderful guide on how simple lifestyle changes can set a person on the course to living a more sustainable and planet-conscious life. Better yet, Stephanie shows readers how to become a sustainability champion in their own households, family, and broader community.

Councilmember Mary M. Cheh, Ward 3 Councilmember on the Council of the District of Columbia

When you enable people and organizations to prioritize the planet and live their values, everybody wins. Individual actions add up. Stephanie Miller wants you to be part of the solution.

Jeremy Brosowsky, Founder, Compost Cab

Stephanie Miller has been a self-aware citizen of Planet Earth. This book is a very readable personal and practical guide to reducing our individual carbon footprint. Stephanie combines facts, science and a very doable recipe for each of us to make a difference to the planet we inhabit. If there is one inheritance we want to leave for our children and grandchildren - it is described in this book in a most user friendly way.

Anita Marangoly George, Executive Vice President, Caisse de dépôt et placement du Québec (CDPQ) and ex- Senior Director for Energy at the World Bank Group

Unlike other books that make going zero waste feel daunting for the average person, *Zero Waste Living, the 80/20 Way*, is the hand-holding equivalent of a friend coaching you through the process offering practical suggestions to modify behavior. The information is accessible, easy to digest, and best of all it is offered in a nonjudgmental way. This should be a first read for anyone interested in making a change to reduce their carbon and plastic footprint. It's also a great read for anyone who has tried but failed to go "cold turkey" in getting to zero waste.

Lara Ilao, Founder of Plastic Tree and Chair of the Circular Economy Working Group

This is the book we have been waiting for. Stephanie connects the dots between the small choices we make every single day as consumers and the global climate challenge. She provides practical actions that even the busiest among us can take to make a difference. **Wendy Teleki**, Head of Women Entrepreneurs Finance Initiative (We-Fi) Secretariat Housed at the World Bank

The world confronts overlapping crises of natural resource depletion, biodiversity loss, pollution of land and sea, and relentless climate change. We can't wait for dithering politicians to take the bold actions required to arrest the destruction of our natural world. In *Zero Waste Living*, Stephanie Miller shows convincingly that you, the reader, can take meaningful actions to help end our unsustainable way of life. Read the book, and be inspired to make a change.
Bart W. Édes, North American Representative, Asian Development Bank and author of *We Should have Seen it Coming*

Resetting Our Future

Zero Waste Living, the 80/20 Way

The Busy Person's Guide to a Lighter Footprint

RESETTING OUR FUTURE

Zero Waste Living, the 80/20 Way

The Busy Person's Guide to a Lighter Footprint

Stephanie J. Miller

CHANGEMAKERS
BOOKS

Winchester, UK
Washington, USA

JOHN HUNT PUBLISHING

First published by Changemakers Books, 2021
Changemakers Books is an imprint of John Hunt Publishing Ltd., No. 3 East Street,
Alresford, Hampshire SO24 9EE, UK
office@jhpbooks.com
www.johnhuntpublishing.com
www.changemakers-books.com

For distributor details and how to order please visit the 'Ordering' section on our website.

ISBN: 978 1 78904 739 4
978 1 78904 740 0 (ebook)
Library of Congress Control Number: 2020945943

A CIP catalogue record for this book is available from the British Library.

Design: Stuart Davies

UK: Printed and bound by CPI Group (UK) Ltd, Croydon, CR0 4YY
Printed in North America by CPI GPS partners

We operate a distinctive and ethical publishing philosophy in
all areas of our business, from our global network of authors to
production and worldwide distribution.

Contents

The *Resetting Our Future* Series

At this critical moment of history, with a pandemic raging, we have the rare opportunity for a Great Reset – to choose a different future. This series provides a platform for pragmatic thought leaders to share their vision for change based on their deep expertise. For communities and nations struggling to cope with the crisis, these books will provide a burst of hope and energy to help us take the first difficult steps towards a better future.
– Tim Ward, publisher, Changemakers Books

What if Solving the Climate Crisis Is Simple?
Tom Bowman, President of Bowman Change, Inc., and Writing Team Lead for the U.S. ACE National Strategic Planning Framework

Zero Waste Living, the 80/20 Way
The Busy Person's Guide to a Lighter Footprint
Stephanie Miller, Founder of Zero Waste in DC, and former Director, IFC Climate Business Department.

A Chicken Can't Lay a Duck Egg
How COVID-19 can Solve the Climate Crisis
Graeme Maxton, (former Secretary-General of the Club of Rome), and Bernice Maxton-Lee (former Director, Jane Goodall Institute)

A Global Playbook for the Next Pandemic
Anne Kabagambe, World Bank Executive Director

Learning from Tomorrow
Using Strategic Foresight to Prepare for the Next Big Disruption
Bart Édes, North American Representative, Asian Development Bank

Impact ED
How Community College Entrepreneurship Programs Create
Prosperity for All
Rebecca Corbin (President, National Association of Community
College Entrepreneurship), Andrew Gold and Mary-Beth Kerly
(both business faculty, Hillsborough Community College).

Power Switch
How We Can Reverse Extreme Inequality
Paul O'Brien, VP, Policy and Advocacy, Oxfam America

SMART Futures for a Sustainable World
Creating a Paradigm Shift for Achieving the Global SDGs
Dr. Claire Nelson, Chief Visionary Officer and Lead Futurist,
The Futures Forum

Reconstructing Blackness
Rev. Charles Howard, Chaplin, University of
Pennsylvania, Philadelphia.

Cut Super Climate Pollutants, Now!
The Ozone Treaty's Urgent Lessons for Speeding up Climate Action
Alan Miller (former World Bank representative for global
climate negotiations) and Durwood Zaelke, (President, The
Institute for Governance & Sustainable Development, and
co-director, The Program on Governance for Sustainable
Development at UC Santa Barbara)

www.ResettingOurFuture.com

For my grandmother, Rosa, the first conservationist
in my life

and

For my mother and father, Marlene and Leonard, who
always made me believe I could do anything I set my
mind to

Foreword

by Thomas Lovejoy

The Pandemic has changed our world. Lives have been lost. Livelihoods as well. Far too many face urgent problems of health and economic security, but almost all of us are reinventing our lives in one way or another. Meeting the immediate needs of the less fortunate is obviously a priority, and a big one. But beyond those compassionate imperatives, there is also tremendous opportunity for what some people are calling a "Great Reset." This series of books, *Resetting Our Future*, is designed to provide pragmatic visionary ideas and stimulate a fundamental rethink of the future of humanity, nature and the economy.

I find myself thinking about my parents, who had lived through the Second World War and the Great Depression, and am still impressed by the sense of frugality they had attained. When packages arrived in the mail, my father would save the paper and string; he did it so systematically I don't recall our ever having to buy string. Our diets were more careful: whether it could be afforded or not, beef was restricted to once a week. When aluminum foil – the great boon to the kitchen – appeared, we used and washed it repeatedly until it fell apart. Bottles, whether coca cola or milk, were recycled.

Waste was consciously avoided. My childhood task was to put out the trash; what goes out of my backdoor today is an unnecessary multiple of that. At least some of it now goes to recycling but a lot more should surely be possible.

There was also a widespread sense of service to a larger community. Military service was required of all. But there was also the Civilian Conservation Corps, which had provided jobs and repaired the ecological destruction that had generated the

1

Dust Bowl. The Kennedy administration introduced the Peace Corps and the President's phrase "Ask not what your country can do for you but what you can do for your country" still resonates in our minds.

There had been antecedents, but in the 1970s there was a global awakening about a growing environmental crisis. In 1972, The United Nations held its first conference on the environment at Stockholm. Most of the modern US institutions and laws about environment were established under moderate Republican administrations (Nixon and Ford). Environment was seen not just as appealing to "greenies" but also as a thoughtful conservative's issue. The largest meeting of Heads of State in history, The Earth Summit, took place in Rio de Janeiro in 1992 and three international conventions – climate change, biodiversity (on which I was consulted) and desertification – came into existence.

But three things changed. First, there now are three times as many people alive today as when I was born and each new person deserves a minimum quality of life. Second, the sense of frugality was succeeded by a growing appetite for affluence and an overall attitude of entitlement. And third, conservative political advisors found advantage in demonizing the environment as comity vanished from the political dialogue.

Insufficient progress has brought humanity and the environment to a crisis state. The CO2 level in the atmosphere at 415 ppm (parts per million) is way beyond a non-disruptive level around 350 ppm. (The pre-industrial level was 280 ppm.)

Human impacts on nature and biodiversity are not just confined to climate change. Those impacts will not produce just a long slide of continuous degradation. The Pandemic is a direct result of intrusion upon, and destruction of, nature as well as wild-animal trade and markets. The scientific body of the UN Convention on Biological Diversity warned in 2020 that we could lose a million species unless there are major changes in human interactions with nature.

We still can turn those situations around. Ecosystem restoration at scale could pull carbon back out of the atmosphere for a soft landing at 1.5 degrees of warming (at 350 ppm), hand in hand with a rapid halt in production and use of fossil fuels. The Amazon tipping point where its hydrological cycle would fail to provide enough rain to maintain the forest in southern and eastern Amazonia can be solved with major reforestation. The oceans' biology is struggling with increasing acidity, warming and ubiquitous pollution with plastics: addressing climate change can lower the first two and efforts to remove plastics from our waste stream can improve the latter.

Indisputably, we need a major reset in our economies, what we produce, and what we consume. We exist on an amazing living planet, with a biological profusion that can provide humanity a cornucopia of benefits—and more that science has yet to reveal—and all of it is automatically recyclable because nature is very good at that. Scientists have determined that we can, in fact, feed all the people on the planet, and the couple billion more who may come, by a combination of selective improvements of productivity, eliminating food waste and altering our diets (which our doctors have been advising us to do anyway).

The *Resetting Our Future* series is intended to help people think about various ways of economic and social rebuilding that will support humanity for the long term. There is no single way to do this and there is plenty of room for creativity in the process, but nature with its capacity for recovery and for recycling can provide us with much inspiration, including ways beyond our current ability to imagine.

Ecosystems do recover from shocks, but the bigger the shock, the more complicated recovery can be. At the end of the Cretaceous period (66 million years ago) a gigantic meteor slammed into the Caribbean near the Yucatan and threw up so much dust and debris into the atmosphere that much of biodiversity perished. It was *sayonara* for the dinosaurs; their only surviving close relatives were precursors to modern day birds. It certainly was not a good time for life on Earth.

The clear lesson of the pandemic is that it makes no sense to generate a global crisis and then hope for a miracle. We are lucky to have the pandemic help us reset our relation to the Living Planet as a whole. We already have building blocks like the United Nations Sustainable Development Goals and various environmental Conventions to help us think through more effective goals and targets. The imperative is to rebuild with humility and imagination, while always conscious of the health of the living planet on which we have the joy and privilege to exist.

Dr. Thomas E. Lovejoy is Professor of Environmental Science and Policy at George Mason University and a Senior Fellow at the United Nations Foundation. A world-renowned conservation biologist, Dr. Lovejoy introduced the term "biological diversity" to the scientific community.

Acknowledgements

I thought that writing a book in less than two months was a challenge, but it turns out that finding the right way to thank all those that made it possible is quite another one altogether.

Let me start by thanking those who found the time to share their perspective with me over the past two months, helping shape my thinking for this book. Anne-Marie Bonneau, Linda Bilsens Brolis, Jeremy Brosowsky, Tony Brusco, D.C. Councilmember Mary Cheh, Charlotte Dreizen, Teresa Erickson, Chad Frischmann, Nora Goldstein, Miranda Gorman, Stephanie Hicks, Prashant Kapoor, Lara Ilao, Matthew Krupp, Mamta Mehra, Victoria Mills, Marcene Mitchell, Gloria Monick, Pete Pearson, Catherine Plume, Beth Porter, Sarah Raposa, Samu Salo, Gaby Seltzer, Erin Simon, Tina Soldovieri, Wendy Teleki, Tom Szaky, Diogo Veríssimo and Kelly Whittier.

I am also indebted for all the support I received from countless colleagues at IFC. It would take another whole book to name them all so I will only mention four by name: my first boss, Dimitris Tsitsiragos, who supported my "green" efforts, even when the ideas themselves were still green; Nena Stoiljkovic, who always understood my passion for environmental issues; and Anita George and Sujoy Bose, friends from near the beginning who supported me through thick and thin. I am grateful to my colleagues in the Climate Business Department, and later the Western Europe team, who worked alongside me to help put climate change at the forefront of our development goals.

Writing my first book has not been a lonely endeavor as I have been blessed with the fellowship of other authors in this series. My friend and fellow author, Paul O'Brien, provided encouragement (and competition) early on to get me past the initial writer's block. Tom Bowman reached the finish line first among my fellow authors and then reached out to help me with my cover design. Special thanks to Melanie Choukas-Bradley, who has provided me with guidance and support along the way. For nearly three decades, I have admired the clarity of Tom Lovejoy's voice as an advocate for the environment, and I am honored that he wrote the forward for our series. I am so grateful to Tim Ward, publisher of Changemakers Books, who trusted my ideas enough to invite me to write this book and who provided just the right mix of encouragement and push to make it happen.

I am blessed by a tight-knit group of friends in the D.C. area who walk—literally and figuratively—alongside me, who cheer me on, who keep me honest and bring joy to my daily life. The Anderson/Volynets's, Campbell/O'Briens, Moloney/Johnstons, Morton/Shtuhls, Brigid Holleran, Stallard/Wilders, Garzonny/Jochnicks, Tudor/Mullens. And a very special mention of two friends who made this book possible: Raquel Gomes, a writer of beautiful non-fiction, who has a masterful eye for editing, helped me see where I needed more or less to help the reader; and Kath Campbell, who joined me early on in my zero waste efforts, nudged me to be bolder and made the "gap year" a lot of fun. Oh, how grateful I am for my friends, near and far.

I wish to thank my wonderful family: Roberta and Steven Miller, the uncle and aunt everyone wishes they had; Cindy and Chris Stephens and their whole brood for their boundless energy and love, and to Cindy in particular for editing the manuscript with the care only a sister could give; my loving brother, Andy Miller; and my mother, Marlene Miller, one of the best writers I know. Finally I am grateful for two people in my daily life: my partner, Matt, who provides unwavering support through all my endeavors and helps me see the blue sky in every day; and for my son, Daniel, who has always brought me so much joy.

Chapter 1

The Aha Moment

We don't need a handful of people doing zero waste perfectly. We need millions of people doing it imperfectly.
Anne-Marie Bonneau, Zero Waste Chef

Big Ideas

I have always been inspired by big ideas. Mitigating climate change. Reducing poverty. Empowering women in developing countries. The process of bringing these big ideas to life, with real and sustainable impact through practical action, has been a driving force for me.

Over the course of 25 years at the International Finance Corporation (IFC), the largest global development institution dedicated to the private sector, I had the privilege of leading climate change mitigation efforts for more than a decade. Eventually I landed my dream job as the director of the then-newly formed Climate Business department, focused on devising climate solutions for our clientele of industry and foreign governments.

During this time, I led the development of a new line of business for IFC in the area of "green buildings," promoting investments in more energy and water efficient buildings. Within three years, this business grew to be one of the biggest climate success stories in the organization. In the process, I embraced the non-purist approach—focused on ambitious but achievable solutions, rather than perfect results—to solving big problems. Let me explain what I mean.

I first worked with a small team to assess the greenhouse gas impact of our investments in some of our key sectors, such as tourism, retail, and commercial property. We realized that we had not looked at the carbon impact of the buildings we were financing in emerging markets, a missed opportunity since buildings account for 20 percent of greenhouse gas emissions and consume 40 percent of global electricity. My boss at the time agreed to let me hire an architect specialized in sustainability. With Prashant Kapoor on board, we worked for months trying to convince investment teams to include him in their project appraisal visits so that he could assess the green buildings potential of these projects.

One team working on a shopping mall investment in Malawi finally reluctantly agreed to let Prashant join the appraisal. During the appraisal, the client's eyes lit up when Prashant explained the energy, water, and cost savings embedded in "green" design choices, things like energy efficient lighting, skylights over shops to reduce the need for artificial lighting, and roof insulation to reduce the demand for air conditioning. These up-front investments would more than pay for themselves in the ensuing several years through energy cost savings. Within months of this appraisal, Prashant became a hot commodity in our organization and was requested on practically all project appraisals involving building construction.

Clients soon began asking for a visible acknowledgment of their green buildings, something their customers and other financiers could easily appreciate. This led us to the design of a standard which, in turn, formed the basis of a certification program we called EDGE: Excellence in Design for Greater Efficiency. (If you are familiar with the U.S. LEED system— Leadership in Energy and Environmental Design—this was a similar notion, but much more practical, inexpensive and therefore accessible for our emerging markets clients.) To qualify for the EDGE certification, buildings would have to meet a threshold of 20 percent increased efficiency in energy and water use, compared with local averages. Our green buildings program eventually became a $6 billion business for IFC.

This story reinforced my belief in how big change can be rooted in pragmatic, people (client)-centered solutions. When we were devising the standard, colleagues at IFC asked: Why only a 20 percent increase in efficiency? Why not 30 or 50 percent? The answer: we wanted to find a threshold that was ambitious but achievable and would quickly create a new market concept. Based on the demand among IFC's clients and now other emerging market players, we think we hit the sweet spot.

* * *

After leaving IFC, my questioning shifted from the sustainable development possibilities at the business and government levels to the resource implications of my own everyday decisions and behaviors. I wondered how I could have more of an impact—or actually, less of an impact—by reducing my personal carbon and waste footprint. What can we—as individuals—do to reverse the current climate and waste crises? Could individual actions have a ripple effect that could lead to systemic change? If so, how could busy people contribute to making these systemic changes?

This book strives to answer these questions and, more importantly, provides practical steps we can all take to make a difference.

A Funny Little Thing

It all started shortly after my farewell party almost two years ago as I left IFC. My 16-year-old son, Daniel, gave a hilarious, surprise speech at the podium and my colleagues' words warmed my heart.

After a long and intense career at IFC, I was burnt out and wanted to spend more time with my son before he headed off to college the following year. So, I took a "gap year" before embarking on my next endeavor. With time on my hands, I signed up for yoga and Pilates classes, met friends for long lunches, cooked more homemade meals, and drove my son to and from school, a luxury working parents rarely have.

And I did a funny, little thing I had been meaning to do for years. I asked the clerk at my local drycleaners if I could bring in a reusable garment bag and have her place our cleaned clothes in there instead of using plastic wrap. The huge amounts of plastic wrap had always bothered me and seemed so unnecessary, but (amazingly) I never found time to make this simple request. "No problem," she said. I left with a huge smile and sense of accomplishment.

During the course of the next week, I did a lot of thinking... what if others like me would love to avoid the plastic, but they are too busy to do anything about it? Is there a way this could be made easier for them?

A quick online search revealed there was such a thing as reusable garment bags specifically for use at the drycleaners. I approached the owner of the drycleaners, Yoon, whom I've known by name for a decade, and asked whether she would consider offering this to her clients. I was prepared to give her data on the cost of the bag and my own sense of the "market" among her clientele. To my surprise, she didn't need any data and embraced the idea, agreeing immediately to order some bags through her wholesale catalog. Again, I left smiling.

This was too easy, I thought. And I was right. Enter Yoon's husband, Ki. The next few times I stopped at the cleaners and enquired about the bags, I got a lot of hemming and hawing, and if Ki was at the counter, a lot of grimaces. It turned out Ki, a savvy businessman, was reluctant to spend the money up-front to purchase the bags without knowing whether clients would actually buy them. Yoon finally got him to agree to order a box of 20. A family friend, Iona, agreed to make a flyer that I posted around town, and I let people on my neighborhood listserv know that these bags were on offer.

Over the next few months, every time I entered the cleaners

(only to drop off my partner's suits as I was spending my life in gym clothes), I would be greeted warmly by Ki and Yoon and a common refrain: "Our customers really love these bags." As of the time of this writing, they have sold more than 360 bags and one third of their customers use them on a regular basis.

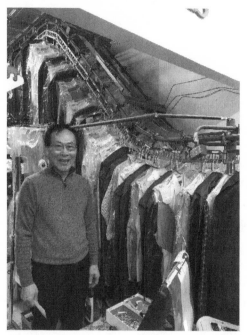

Ki at President Valet. Photo by Stephanie Miller.

I encouraged friends to ask their cleaners to offer the same thing, with limited success (so far). But what this showed me very clearly was three things:

1. busy people may want to do the right thing, but just don't have time,
2. businesses may want to do the right thing, but fear taking a risk that will affect their bottom line, and
3. once people see a new, easy way they can do the right thing, they jump pretty quickly on the bandwagon.

At about the same time, my friend Wendy—on hearing about my drycleaning escapades—suggested I might enjoy reading Bea Johnson's *A Zero Waste Home*. She spoke about the ideas in the book passionately: "My daughter and I were so excited about the concept that we spent the weekend re-arranging everything in our kitchen." This is how I was introduced to the concept of zero waste living.

What Is Zero Waste Living?

Zero waste living is a movement that promotes less consumption and less waste. The goal is to reduce trash, particularly what we send to landfills, incinerators, and the ocean. Zero waste living embraces the concept of "Reduce, Reuse, Recycle," but takes this waste hierarchy to a completely different level.

Drastically reducing our consumption is the first step: the less we buy, the less we waste. Our convenience culture has made this difficult, but not impossible. Most zero waste books will have you analyze your waste stream so that you gain a better understanding of your family's consumption patterns. These books will also show you alternatives in every room of your home—starting with the kitchen—for how to reduce waste and find reusable or less wasteful alternatives. For example, most of us consider paper towels to be a staple, but they can easily be replaced by reusable washcloths. In the bathroom, we might be using disposable plastic razors, but we could use safety razors instead. Zero waste living means that you shop differently, cook differently and even travel differently. There are literally *thousands of things* an individual can do to reduce his or her waste at home and at work.

Zero waste experts will admit that you can never really get to zero waste, as our society does not make this possible. Even if you purchase something in the bulk section of a store— say, cashews—that product had to be transported from the producer to the grocer in a container that was most likely plastic.

Nonetheless, the problem is additive, and consumers account for a significant part of the plastics waste stream so their actions can make a big difference.

What I love about the zero waste concept is that it intersects nicely with so many other agendas aimed at reducing an individual's footprint: minimalism (think Marie Kondo, author of *The Life-Changing Magic of Tidying Up*); the effort to save the oceans and marine life from plastics and other pollutants; the environmental movement; the shift to relying on a second-hand economy (lower your consumption by using or repairing what already exists); the circular economy movement (based on the idea of designing out waste; the opposite of a linear economy, which uses and then disposes of resources); and the push to support our local economy (patronize small local businesses and reduce the need for goods to travel long distances). And, for me, the connection with climate change is crystal clear: the less you consume and throw away, the more energy is saved, which results in fewer greenhouse gas emissions.

Almost immediately after reading Bea Johnson, I embarked with gusto on my quest to get to zero waste.

My Personal Experiment

Thank goodness I was taking a gap year. As I read Bea Johnson's book and those of other experts, I realized that getting to zero waste was going to take a lot of time out of my day. Johnson provides recipes for laundry detergent, mascara, shampoo, insect repellent and even a recipe for making your own paper. I was intrigued. I was motivated. And at least at first, I was undaunted. The image of the end goal is well known in the zero waste community: an entire year of trash fitting into a mason jar. It would be worth the effort.

Now, I am not what you would call a do-it-yourself kind of person, so I did not rush things. But I did start to look for opportunities to make things from scratch—e.g., homemade granola (see box below), vegetable broth and cotton produce bags — and to buy items that came in less packaging. I did finally manage to make my own household cleaner, but making lip balm remains on my to-do list.

The Cereal Dilemma

The first week I posted about my zero waste efforts on social media, I proudly showed off my recycle bins from one week to the next. I was happily surprised by how quickly we cut our recycling waste in half.

Not quite zero waste though. Remnants in that second bin: seven cans of dog food, beer bottles, a carton of half and half, a pasta box, a plastic clamshell for raspberries, three boxes of cereal.

Three boxes of cereal? Only one of us in the house ate cereal that week, my partner, Matt.

Intent on making more progress towards reducing waste, I approached Matt about the cereal. Would he be willing to try granola from bulk bins to avoid the packaging? "No," he replied, politely. Cracklin' Oat Bran was something he had really relished since childhood. He loved it so much that, when he was living overseas, he'd always managed to pack a few boxes in his suitcase when he visited the U.S. Hmm. Would he be willing to try homemade granola? "Well, maybe." But just to reduce the quantity of cereal boxes a bit, not eliminate them completely. I still hoped we could get to zero waste, but I realized this would not be as easy as I had first thought.

At the same time as I was moving slowly towards my zero waste goals, I started talking to as many people as I could about subjects that touched on zero waste and/or climate change mitigation. Tapping into my former network and branching out into new areas, I found experts on a range of subjects: home solar installation, composting, recycling, food waste and plastics. I visited recycling plants in my region and I started a regular dialogue with my city's recycling office about questions I had. I discovered the joys of composting. I learned about the fascinating and flawed aspects of recycling systems. I found out how food waste is a factor in greenhouse gas emissions and that individual households are a significant contributor to the problem. I discovered that it made no sense to install solar panels on our roof as the shade of our beautiful oak tree blocked all the sun; and solar technology—though much improved over the past two decades—could still not detect sunshine through the shade of a thick tree. I started noticing how much money I was saving (a lot, and very welcome during my gap year which was accompanied by a big gap in income) by buying less, buying in bulk, and making do with what we had on hand. I watched documentaries with names like *The Story of Plastic* and *Trash Empire*.

With respect to plastics, I began to notice plastic packaging. It was as if I had been previously blinded to plastic and then suddenly, there it was, *everywhere*. Here is an example of what I mean: shortly after embarking on this journey, I went to a favorite local butcher, intent on buying my chicken at the deli counter using my own container. As I walked into the shop and made my way to the counter, I noticed the island of products on offer between the cashier and the deli counter: *every single item* had been re-packaged into small or medium plastic clamshell containers. Nuts, dried fruit, homemade baked goods, candies. By shelf space, these items took up most of the store. Was I the only one who was seeing this? Surely, the other customers must notice this sea of plastic. But when I looked around, nobody seemed fazed.

Shortly thereafter, I had similar experiences at Safeway and

Whole Foods. I did what my zero waste books suggested: I shopped on the perimeter of the store in the fresh produce aisles and brought my own reusable bags for bagging loose vegetables and fruit. When I got to the register to pay, I assumed there would be others relying on reusable bags for their fresh produce. Not a soul. My world seemed to be different from the one occupied by everyone around me. Of course, this wasn't true, but I would have to shop in different places—like the nearby Takoma Park Silver Spring Food Co-op, with its wide variety of bulk food options—to find kindred spirits.

In fact, I soon discovered there are many kindred spirits. An initiative called Plastic Free July (www.plasticfreejuly.org), for example, counts more than 326 million people across the globe who signed up to the challenge in July 2020 to reduce their household waste. But I wondered what it would take for more people to be willing to make changes to reduce their footprint.

The *80/20* Rule

I was eager to be a perfect zero waster, but as the end of my gap year neared, my mason jar of trash remained but a vision.

When we are trying to solve a difficult problem, we tend to look to what worked for us in the past. That's when I had my aha moment: a simple rule that guided me in the world of business and economics could serve me here, too. It's the 80/20 rule, also called the *Pareto Principle*, that says the majority of results are often caused by only a few actions. It's often the case, for example, that 80 percent of business comes from 20 percent of clients. Any good human resources professional will tell you that 80 percent of your time as a manager is spent with 20 percent of staff (usually the highest and lowest performers). It doesn't have to be exact, but it serves as a good guiding principle to try to identify the most significant actions that could make the biggest difference.

What was the 80/20 rule for zero waste? I asked myself.

Luckily, I stumbled on an inspiring book, a compilation really: Paul Hawken's *Drawdown: The Most Comprehensive Plan Ever Proposed to Reverse Global Warming*. In it, Hawken assembles an international coalition of scientists and researchers to offer a list of 80 solutions—all viable—that if taken collectively, would reverse climate change. Bingo: this is what would help me find the 80/20 actions that would guide my zero waste efforts.

Hawken describes actions that need to be taken by national governments, municipalities, industry, consumer-facing businesses, and individuals to slow and even reverse the current global warming trends, ranked by their potential impact. The first two most impactful actions are the safe disposal of chemical refrigerants (the stuff in our refrigerators and A/C systems) and the installation of onshore wind turbines. Decisions that we can influence as individual voters and consumers, but that require direct action by governments and industry. However, the third and fourth items on the list—reducing food waste and adopting a plant-rich diet—most definitely fall partly or mostly within the domain of the individual. Adopting a plant-rich diet is almost entirely an individual choice. Sustainably addressing food waste requires action by governments and businesses, but also by individuals as households account for more than 40 percent of all the food waste in the United States.

As I went down the list, I noticed there were plenty of other steps that individuals could take to reduce their carbon footprint, but I also realized many of them would be difficult— time consuming or expensive—to undertake. Rooftop solar, for example, number ten on the list, can result in great energy and cost savings over time, but requires an up-front investment beyond the financial reach of many. Electric vehicles and electric bikes are two other proposed solutions on the list, but can also be prohibitively expensive, or in the case of electric bikes, not viable for large segments of the population.

Armed with the knowledge from *Drawdown*, my many

conversations with experts, and my own personal experience over the course of what ended up being an 18-month gap "year," I realized I now had what I needed to figure out the 80/20 rule for zero waste living. The key actions around zero waste needed to meet two requirements: they each needed to be highly impactful from a carbon and/or waste reduction perspective *and* they needed to be easy to implement. I came up with ten action steps that fit these criteria and I realized these actions fell within three themes: focus on food, purge plastics and recycle right, my "magic three." These themes and the actions around them became my guiding principles for zero waste living the 80/20 way.

* * *

Let me be clear. The climate and waste crises must be tackled by all three actors: governments, private sector and individuals. I am in no way absolving governments and industry from doing their part and, in fact, those two actors have the most to do. But individuals can do more than they imagine. Beyond reducing our own footprint, our actions can spur new social norms and, collectively, they can signal what we expect from businesses vying for our dollars and elected officials vying for our votes.

The Magic Three

This book is structured around the Magic Three — focus on food, purge plastics and recycle right. Each of the next three chapters will focus on one of these themes. In them, I synthesize the science behind each theme and offer specific actions that meet the 80/20 test: they must be easy to implement and make a big difference. There are only ten action steps that I am suggesting are critical. They are not all equally easy, but all are worth the effort.

In the last chapter, we'll explore how you can promote changes beyond your household, while still keeping your day job.

As I write, we are in the midst of the coronavirus pandemic that is ravaging communities and our economy. One possible silver lining, at least for those of us who are privileged enough to have some extra time, is that the pandemic has forced us to slow down and rethink how we go about shopping for food, traveling, working, and studying. Already we have drastically altered patterns of behavior and consumption that were unthinkable a few months ago. For example, the business models for our food supply have had to shift overnight. Pete Pearson, Senior Director for Food Waste at the World Wildlife Fund, calls this "the great re-configuration," as grocery stores and other suppliers have switched their way of doing business to accommodate the new demand for online shopping and delivery. Another example is air travel: will we ever go back to "business as usual," where we hop on a plane for a one-day meeting now that we've seen how much can be accomplished with virtual meetings?

Much like my gap year, the pandemic can be viewed as an opportunity to step back from the "noise" of a busy daily life to imagine possibilities. And very much like my gap year, the pandemic gives us perhaps a once-in-a-lifetime chance to reframe how we want to live in this world. Just as the pandemic has forced us to rethink our behaviors, the climate and waste crises urge us to do the same. This book offers some steps in that direction.

Chapter 2

Focus on Food

Eat food. Mostly plants. Not too much.
Michael Pollan

Despite a career immersed in climate change issues, my biggest surprises when I embarked on my zero waste journey were not around plastic waste or recycling. They were all around food.

Here are some statistics that got my attention:

- *If global food waste were a country, it would be the third largest emitter of greenhouse gases* after the U.S. and China.[1] Food waste is a direct contributor to climate change because of greenhouse gas emissions: 8 percent in total. That's... well... huge.
- *Household-level food waste is highest in the U.S., with Americans wasting 43 percent of food brought into our homes.*[2] This makes households the single largest source of food waste in the U.S., even ahead of consumer-facing businesses like grocery stores. Lots we can do about this.
- *Livestock are the leading source of greenhouse gas emissions*, at 14.5 percent of the world's total.[3] Not surprisingly, then, becoming a vegetarian is the single most impactful thing we can do as individuals to reduce our carbon footprint.
- *Food that ends up in landfills produces tons of methane and landfills are the third largest source of methane emissions in the U.S.*[4] Methane is a gas at least 28 times more powerful than carbon dioxide at trapping the earth's heat over a 20-year time horizon.[5] By contrast, food

waste that is composted is exposed to oxygen and the decomposition process results in carbon dioxide instead of methane emissions. Much better, right? That's exactly how I felt.

The 80/20 Food Plan

When I looked closely at what I could do that was manageable *and* impactful in reducing my carbon footprint, I realized there were three obvious areas I needed to tackle: increase plant-based meals in my diet, reduce my food waste, and start composting.

Plant-Based Diet

In 2009, IFC sent me to England to attend a sustainability learning workshop offered by Cambridge University. I learned about the latest thinking on climate change, the greenhouse gas contribution of some of the key sectors that we were financing, and ways we might mitigate the impact of these investments. I got to visit one of the Cambridge laboratories to see ice core cylinders drilled deep out of the Antarctic ice sheet, with air bubbles dating back 800,000 years that provide researchers a window into atmospheric changes over millennia. It was mesmerizing.

Yet perhaps most surprising was the session on how meat-based diets contribute to man-made global warming. If cattle were a country, they would be the third-largest emitter of greenhouse gases.[6] I had been oblivious up to that point. I remember feeling shocked that we were given this data one afternoon and then were served bacon for breakfast in the cafeteria the following morning. If I were ever to become a vegetarian, that was the week it should have happened.

The importance of plant-rich diets is now well known. Maybe you have been inspired to eat a bit less meat after reading Michael Pollan's *The Omnivore's Dilemma*. Or maybe your doctor suggested cutting down on meat and dairy to improve your cholesterol. Maybe you have already made some little shifts in your diet. Or maybe you haven't.

The good news for those of us who have not taken the plunge to becoming full-fledged vegetarians is that we can make a difference even by shifting our consumption habits just a bit. Consider the data: a 2019 study in Scientific Reports[7] concluded that if everyone in the U.S. substituted plant proteins for meat proteins 25 percent of the time, we would reduce annual greenhouse gas emissions by 82 million tons, a bit more than one percent a year. This may sound like nothing, but it is equivalent to taking about 18 million cars off the road every year.

I was also inspired by Jonathan Safran Foer's *We Are the Weather: Saving the Planet Begins at Breakfast*, which makes the compelling, empirically sound argument that we can't solve the climate crisis without addressing animal agriculture. Foer's call: "Everyone will eat a meal relatively soon and can immediately participate in the reversal of climate change." Interestingly, Foer does not advocate for going vegetarian, but rather eliminating animal products at breakfast and lunch. This is a relatively painless step individuals can take and know they are making a significant dent in the problem.

Enter the 80/20 rule…I committed to reduce my meat-based meals by 25 percent, a relatively small step that would make a big difference in my personal carbon impact.

Action Step: Go part-vegetarian (vegetarians, please feel free to skip to the next section)

As it turns out, most of my breakfasts and many of my lunches are meatless, so reaching the 25 percent more plant-based meals threshold meant tackling the near-sacred notion in our household that dinner was not really dinner if meat were not the centerpiece. My goal was to move towards three square vegetarian dinners every week.

I decided a big announcement to the family was not necessary.

Instead, I looked up the best vegetarian recipes I could find that seemed relatively simple and started introducing these once a week. I began with vegetarian recipes from trusted cookbooks. *Milk Street Tuesday Nights* (thanks, Megan, for the gift that keeps on giving) has a great recipe for Turkish Red Lentil Soup and another for White Beans with Sage, Garlic and Fennel. Both were big hits at our dinner table.

Next, I moved on to Ottolenghi's *Plenty* (a birthday gift from my mother) and later *Plenty More*, both vegetarian cookbooks. There's quite a bit of work involved in most Ottolenghi recipes, I find. And some of the ingredients can be hard to track down. Some days it's worth it, and some days it is just too much work for a weeknight meal. I will save you the time in testing the recipes and tell you the hands-down "keepers" were: Chickpea, Tomato and Bread Soup (I often dream about this one); Tagliatelle with Walnuts and Lemon; and Crushed Puy Lentils with Tahini and Cumin. If I put one of these meals on the table and make enough for leftovers the following night, I only then need to find one more vegetarian meal for the week.

Two friends Brigid and Raquel separately reminded me that Mollie Katzen's Moosewood Cookbook series was their introduction to the world of tasty vegetarian meals, and insist that the Spinach Ricotta Pie is amazing.

The *New York Times Cooking* app has provided more great vegetarian recipe ideas and I like that I can see how other readers/ cooks have rated the recipes. Votes count. Democracy works. How did I survive all these years without Marcella Hazan's famous —and incredibly simple—tomato sauce recipe? Or Mark Bittman's pesto recipe? If I serve either of these up for dinner with pasta nobody even notices that it's a vegetarian meal.

The other advantage of using this app is that I get inspiration for meals that use seasonal ingredients. As my friend Kath says: there's no point cooking a dish with fresh tomatoes if the tomatoes have had to travel more than 2000 miles from Mexico.

This is an important point as the long-haul transport of produce has financial and environmental costs. The tomatoes also lose a lot of their flavor on the long journey. As I write this, it *is* tomato season and I am making gazpacho at least twice a week using local tomatoes, often from our kitchen garden. I have included my favorite gazpacho recipe from my friend and chef Kell in Appendix 2. It is well loved and a winner.

Action Step: Prioritize your diet based on the carbon intensity of food

Not all food is created equal. Some have a heavier carbon footprint than others.

The chart below represents greenhouse gas emissions per

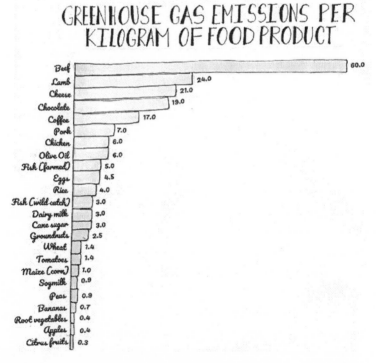

GREENHOUSE GAS EMISSIONS PER KILOGRAM OF FOOD PRODUCT

Food	Emissions
Beef	60.0
Lamb	24.0
Cheese	21.0
Chocolate	19.0
Coffee	17.0
Pork	7.0
Chicken	6.0
Olive Oil	6.0
Fish (farmed)	5.0
Eggs	4.5
Rice	4.0
Fish (wild catch)	3.0
Dairy milk	3.0
Cane sugar	3.0
Groundnuts	2.5
Wheat	1.4
Tomatoes	1.4
Maize (corn)	1.0
Soymilk	0.9
Peas	0.9
Bananas	0.7
Root vegetables	0.4
Apples	0.4
Citrus fruits	0.3

Adapted from *Our World in Data, Environmental Impacts of Food* (2018). Illustration by Iona Volynets.

kilogram of common food items. Not surprisingly, meat leads the pack by a longshot, with 60 kilograms of greenhouse gas for every kilogram of beef.

According to bestselling cookbook author Mark Bittman, "In terms of energy consumption, serving a family-of-four steak dinner is the rough equivalent of driving around in an SUV for three hours while leaving all the lights on at home."[8] That's something you can sink your teeth into.

Now, I'm not always going to have a dinner of peas instead of steak, but noticing that one kilogram of wild-caught fish is responsible for only three kilograms of greenhouse gas emissions makes me quite inclined to order the filet of wild salmon instead of the steak the next time we eat out. I was pained to see the reference data for chocolate and coffee as I am pretty sure I can reduce these only so much in my diet. Consider printing this chart and placing it on your refrigerator until you start to get a good sense of how carbon intensive your food choices are.

Where's the Beyond Beef? An important new trend that is making vegetarian meals a lot more accessible for omnivores is the next generation of meat substitutes. Out of nowhere, it seems, Beyond Beef and the Impossible Burger have arrived on the scene and are infiltrating burger joints like Burger King and White Castle, as well as swankier restaurants. These products are widely available in supermarkets and are an easy substitute for recipes that call for ground beef. In fact, meatless burgers have been around for about a decade but became mainstream once Whole Foods placed them in meat aisles in 2016.

How have these new plant-based meat alternatives broken into a market that had been stagnant for decades? In the case of the Impossible Burger, its "secret sauce" is something called a heme. A heme is an essential molecule that occurs naturally in humans, animals and plants. According to the makers of the Impossible Burger, heme is "what makes meat taste like meat." Somewhat controversially, Impossible Foods has produced genetically modified hemes from fermented soybeans. Questionable process perhaps, but the upside is that this meat product is much more environmentally sustainable. According to the company, the Impossible Burger generates 87 percent less greenhouse gas, requires 95 percent less land, and uses 75 percent less water to produce than beef burgers.[9]

For the sake of research, I ordered a pizza from my local pizza joint this week with a topping of Impossible Burger. It was surprisingly indistinguishable from ground beef and I keep hearing stories from friends about how satisfied (and incredulous) they are when they fry up morning sausages or grill burgers made with these meat substitutes. Here is what my friend Teresa had to say:

> I've tried *every* kind of veggie burger under the sun; they were awful *and* unhealthy – either with too much sodium or too much soy. The first time I had a Beyond Beef burger it felt like a choir of angels was singing above me. It actually tastes like meat! Somehow, they've managed to incorporate that mouthfeel of chopped sirloin marbled with just the right amount of fat. But even better, after a Beyond Beef burger, I don't have that bloated stomach feeling I used to get after a really delicious burger. I use it in everything now – spaghetti sauce, meatballs, lasagna. I should buy stock in it!

Yes, Teresa, you probably should. These brands seem to have stumbled on a magical formula in taste and texture, and this provides yet another vegetarian option to choose from... and just in time to help with the climate crisis.

Handy Tips

Synchronizing expectations at family meals. Your family may eventually catch on to the fact that you have switched out the meat from many of their meals. They may protest. You may try to explain to them why you think it's important for the planet and their health and they may be unconvinced. They may, for example, say: Please, no more than one or two vegetarian meals per week, for goodness' sake. If you find yourself in this situation, do not despair. Make the one to two vegetarian meals for everyone and then eat some of your own meals without the meat. I used to think this was "uncommunal," but it's fine. Really.

Finding time. Whether vegetarian or non-vegetarian meals, the thing most likely to derail us from cooking—especially during the work week—is running low on time or energy. One solution is freezing cooked meals ahead of time. In the weeks before giving birth to my son (18 years ago), I recall I froze many a stew in anticipation of the exhaustion that was likely in those first few weeks. Boy, was I grateful for those stews. We often use our weekends to cook up big batches of recipes and then freeze some portions for mid-week dinners. Meals that freeze particularly well are bean burgers, vegetable soup, lentil soup, vegetarian chili and pasta sauces.

* * *

Food Waste

Reducing food waste is the number three action listed as a way to reverse global warming in Paul Hawken's *Drawdown: The Most Comprehensive Plan Ever Proposed to Reverse Global Warming*.

While some food waste at the household level is unavoidable (think chicken bones and banana peels), most of our household food waste could be reduced through better food planning and management.

Action Step: Food planning

As a consumer, it all starts with what you buy. According to a study by the World Wildlife Fund, 34 percent of Americans rarely or never take stock of their groceries before going to the store.[10]

If we look at the waste hierarchy pictured below, "reduce" is at the top for a reason. In the case of food, there is nothing to waste if you eat exactly what you purchase. Is this hard to do? Yes. Is it impossible? No. Is it easier than flying less on airplanes or never using our cars? Definitely.

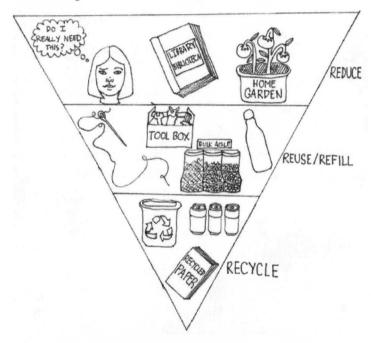

Waste hierarchy. Illustration by Iona Volynets.

This does mean you need to be a conscious buyer. *Plan your meals for the week and never go grocery shopping without a list.*

Pick a day when you (alone, or with your family) decide on meals. Plans change—friends invite you to a last-minute dinner or you are too tired to cook—but you need a plan. Without a plan, you will bring every delicious looking "find" from the store into your home, and you will waste much of it. How do I know? *Because the average American throws away 400 pounds of food per year.*[11]

Here is what I do.

Every Saturday, Matt and I plan the meals for the week. Since I am taking responsibility for the three vegetarian meals, this means I come to the table with three suggestions. Matt suggests another couple of meals. That's a total of five so far. One meal a week is usually takeout (prior to the pandemic it was likely a restaurant meal). And we save one night per week as a "leftovers night." We post these meals on the fridge on an eraser board that allows us to write in one meal for each day of the week. No more questions about "what's for dinner tonight."

Immediately after planning our seven meals, we make a grocery list. This is obviously key and not straying from the list is also critical. How long do the meal plans and grocery list take? About 15–20 minutes.

If you do those two things carefully—meal planning and making your grocery list—you are more than halfway there.

Now we need to tackle the food that enters your home.

Action Step: The daily 3-minute fridge review

Set a time of day—mid-morning after breakfast, right before or right after dinner. Whatever works best for you. Set an alarm if you must and then just do it.

What is my goal during the fridge review?

- Move older foods forward so that they are visible and more likely to be eaten first
- Look for food that is getting moldy. Get it out of the fridge (trash or compost)
- Identify food I need to use immediately

Tricks:

- Create a drawer or shelf for items that should be eaten first. If there are others in your household and they may not know your system by heart, label this shelf or drawer as shown in the picture below.

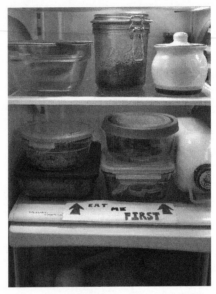

Our fridge. Photo by Stephanie Miller.

- Use see-through containers so that there are no food surprises. I use Pyrex storage bowls or glass jars. The more quickly you (and others) can identify what is in your fridge, the less likely the food item will sit there unnoticed and eventually go bad.
- Use expiration dates as a guide but not the Bible. Rely on your senses (sight, smell, taste) to determine whether something needs to be thrown away.
- Prep veggies as soon as you unpack them. This will later save you valuable time and energy when it is time to cook. Your *future self* will thank you.

Action Step: Use-it-up cooking

Once you know what is in your fridge, you need a strategy for how to use what is there. If you have done your planning, there should not be too many surprises. But you will never perfectly be able to predict what will be eaten when. Here are some things you can do with what you find:

- Have one or two recipes that allow you to mix and match ingredients you have on hand. My go-to recipe is a very simple stir-fry I have adapted from a Mark Bittman recipe.
- One of my favorite zero waste bloggers Anne-Marie Bonneau aka The Zero Waste Chef has a great article (*Avoid the Store a Little Longer: Shop the Refrigerator and Pantry*) in which she offers soup, pizza, chili, dal and other recipes that allow for a lot of ingredient versatility.
- Use cooking apps to find recipes for ingredients you have on hand. I recently started using a helpful app called *Supercook* which provides recipe ideas based on whatever ingredients you list.

Action Step: Schedule a regular leftovers night

I have talked to lots of families who have found this challenging in the past, but easier since the pandemic. I used to hear things like, "My kids refuse to eat leftovers" or "My partner prefers a freshly cooked meal." My friend Wendy who has a family of five says: "Leftovers night is not optional anymore. Everyone—even the kids—just accepts it now."

Action Step: Make your freezer your ally

Use your freezer liberally. I had no idea how many things you can successfully freeze... soup stock, fresh herbs, tomato paste, and even dairy. If I will not finish up the berries before they turn bad, I freeze them. When I have meal leftovers that we will not want to see again for a while, I freeze them. When I squeeze a lemon or lime for the juice I need for a recipe and still have some to spare, I freeze the extra. If you freeze in glass containers, as I often do, be sure to leave some space (an inch or two) between the food and the lid as frozen liquids expand and you do not want to end up with cracked glass. Also be sure to label and date your items before you freeze them. You would be surprised how unrecognizable everything is when it forms into an icy mass and you will have long forgotten what you placed in the container.

But here is the most important thing I can say on this subject: you must freeze food in a timely way. You will not trust your food in the freezer to be edible if you wait too long to freeze it. The three-minute fridge review ensures you are catching things on day three and not day six.

And do not forget to use what is in your freezer. If you are taking the time to freeze more food, you need to make a regular habit of using what's in the freezer. Again, I love Anne-Marie Bonneau's concept for avoiding food waste: shop your freezer, refrigerator and pantry before you hit the store. Every couple of months or so, we'll plan meals for the week based on what we can defrost from our freezer.

* * *

Composting

Truly incredible for me to fathom… how did I not know all these years that food waste in landfills is such a huge contributor to greenhouse gas emissions? Why hadn't anyone told me?

If you are a busy, urban professional looking for a quick win, this is it. Immediate effect from your composting: a substantial drop in your weekly trash volume, which in turn directly reduces emissions from methane, one of the most powerful greenhouse gases.

Action Step: Compost your food scraps

Does this fit the 80/20 rule? Absolutely... it is a highly impactful shift and it is easy to do. If you come from a large urban community, you may have access to the two easiest composting options:

- Compost drop-off points offered by your municipality. In D.C., where I live, there is a drop-off site in each of our eight wards. New York City has the country's largest drop-off program, although this was suspended during the coronavirus pandemic.
- Fee-based residential compost service. In the D.C. region, two comparable companies offer weekly pick-up of your food scraps for $8/week. They also offer two free bags of composted soil to interested customers. Until I started composting in my own backyard more recently, the service I used was Compost Cab, a company that was founded in 2010 and is a pioneer in home pick-up service.

Check out Compost Now (compostnow.org/compost-services/) or Litterless (litterless.com/wheretocompost) to learn if there is a compost drop-off point or doorstep service in your neighborhood. Besides tracking compost options across the U.S. and Canada, Compost Now, a North Carolina-based company, also offers pick-up service in their region and is considering expanding to new locations based on registered waitlist interest on their website.

What should you do if neither drop-off nor pick-up service is available near you? According to Jeremy Brosowsky, founder of Compost Cab, your next best bet is to look for urban farms and community gardens that offer independent drop-off options. The Institute for Local Self-Reliance offers a map to track locations across the U.S. (ilsr.org/composting/map/). You can also google "community composting near me" or "master gardener near me." Master gardeners exist in every state and should be able to guide you on composting options in your community.

Finally, if you cannot find any of the above, consider composting yourself. It is more ambitious, but highly satisfying to install your own compost system, especially if you have a backyard. I finally did this a few months ago (see photo below). A "system" makes this sound like a complex process. In fact, it is very simple: you mix your daily "greens" of vegetable and fruit scraps (e.g., apple cores, carrot peels, even coffee grinds) with "browns" (e.g., dry leaves, shredded paper). Oxygen, heat and moisture combine to break down the organic material. A few months later you end up with what my gardening friend Dawn calls "black gold," the finished compost which can be added to your soil as a natural fertilizer for plants.

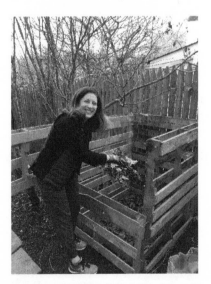

Our backyard compost bin. Photo by Matt Harrington.

My friends Kath and Gerry built me a compost bin in my backyard as a birthday gift last year. They took wooden pallets from a construction site and repurposed them to form the walls and gate of my compost bin. If you want to try to make one of these pallet compost bins, be sure to use ones that are stamped with the "IPPC" or "EPAL" logo, plus the letters HT, which stands for "heat-treated." This ensures there is no risk of toxic materials leaching into your compost. Some pallets have been treated with toxic chemicals that you definitely want to avoid.

The only drawback of home composting is that you may not be able to compost as many materials in your home system. For instance, when I used a pick-up service, I would leave stale bread and rice in the bin for pick-up. These are risky items to put in our backyard system as they can attract rodents.

Even if you live in an apartment, there are compact compost systems available. Vermicomposting (also known as worm composting) is a way to compost indoors using small, red wiggler worms that break down your kitchen scraps into finished compost. I had never heard of this until recently, but there is a plethora of guidance available online.

Nothing on this zero waste journey has been more satisfying to me than when I began composting. Try it and I'm pretty sure you'll agree.

Chapter 3

Purge Plastics

The most environmentally friendly product is the one you didn't buy.
Joshua Becker

Because of the vivid images we have seen of the turtle with a straw lodged in its nostril and Greenpeace's highly effective campaign to bring attention to the ocean plastics crisis, it is easy to make the association between plastics and threats to marine life. This has helped launch the plastic straw ban and compelled some of the largest consumer products companies (think Coca-Cola and Procter & Gamble) to try to address the issue with clean-up efforts and use of more recycled material. But plastics are more than a marine pollution issue. They are also a climate change and a health issue. The shocking data:

- *Plastic production is a significant contributor to climate change.* In 2019, the production and incineration of plastic produced more than 850 million tons of greenhouse gases. Even more shocking is the expectation about future plastic production based on expected demand. On the current trajectory, by 2030 greenhouse gas emissions from plastics could reach 1.3 billion tons per year,[1] equivalent to emissions from about 280 million cars. I knew plastics production was energy intensive, but hadn't realized how much it contributes to greenhouse gas emissions.
- *In 1997, researchers discovered a massive area of plastic waste and other debris in the Pacific Ocean.* The Great Pacific Garbage Patch, as they coined it, covers a surface area that is twice the size of Texas and three times the size

of France. The Great Pacific Garbage Patch is one of five plastic accumulation zones in the world's oceans.[2]

- *Researchers project that by 2050, oceans will have more plastic than fish.*[3] Large plastic breaks down into microplastics... so what you see floating on the ocean is a tiny fraction of what is in the water column and lying on the seabed.[4] 2050 is around the corner: My 18-year-old son will be 48 years old that year. Will he be gazing at a sea of plastic when he goes to the beach?

- *The chemicals industry is planning to invest more than $200 billion in new ethane cracker facilities which will emit hazardous air pollutants.* Ethane cracker plants— the facilities that transform natural gas into the resin that makes plastics—emit benzene, linked to cancer and childhood leukemia; toluene, linked to brain, liver and kidney problems, as well as infant mortality and birth defects; and formaldehyde, a known carcinogen.[5]

A Short History of Single-Use Plastic... because it IS short

Single-use plastic is the stuff that you use once or twice and then you throw away or recycle. This is distinct from multi-use plastic, which is things like plastic crates used again and again by farmers and grocers or medical equipment in hospitals.

Single-use plastic is things like:

- the plastic water bottle you recently bought
- your Starbucks coffee cup (lined with plastic and recyclable in *very few* jurisdictions)
- the disposable gloves you use to protect yourself from the coronavirus
- the plastic utensils you didn't ask for in your last restaurant takeout order
- the containers your food is placed in for your restaurant

takeout order
- the packaging around your toilet paper and paper towels
- the plastic wrap you use to cover your leftovers
- the produce bags you use to shop for your vegetables and fruit
- the clamshell containers that hold the nuts or cookies you recently bought at the grocery store.

Though single use plastic was invented fairly recently—the first plastic shopping bag was patented in 1965 in Sweden—it was only in 1982 that two of the biggest supermarket chains in the U.S., Safeway and Kroger, replaced paper bags with plastic bags. By 2011, one million plastic bags were consumed every minute across the globe.[6]

In short, single-use plastic is packaging that you probably touch for only seconds or minutes before you dispose of it. Because it is ubiquitous and *so* convenient, it takes some effort to avoid. But it is not impossible. It just takes a bit of commitment.

The 80/20 Plastics Plan
Action step: Pick one thing

If you were to invite me into your home and let me spend half an hour there—and assuming you let me peek into your fridge, kitchen cupboards, bathroom and garbage bins—I could quickly identify where your biggest opportunities would be to drastically reduce your single-use plastic. But you probably have a fairly good sense anyway. So, here is my advice: pick the most obvious thing. Pick something you buy regularly and commit to 1) finding the non-plastic alternative and 2) never buying it in plastic again.

For me, the thing I picked was water in plastic bottles. If you buy two plastic water bottles a day (which I often did), then the math is simple: you avoid 730 plastic bottles every year.

When I was going into the office every day, it meant

remembering to bring my own bottle from home. It also meant that if I forgot my bottle, I would drink from water fountains instead and sometimes go a bit thirsty. This helped me remember my bottle the next day. The first time I traveled by plane after making this commitment, I had to remember to empty my bottle before going through security and then refill it after security.

For my friend Sarah it was coffee cups. She committed to only buying take-out coffee with her reusable cup. As head of IFC's corporate responsibility program, she knows the power of transparency for accountability. So she shared her commitment with colleagues. When she found herself at her office coffee shop without her reusable cup on hand, steps from a colleague with whom she had shared her commitment, she promptly turned around and did without coffee. She never forgot her cup again.

In the last chapter on food, I suggested eight action steps. In this chapter, I am only suggesting this one. This is because I am convinced that once you commit to eliminating one of your frequently used plastic items, you will start looking for other opportunities to cut single-use plastic out of your life. And if you have not done so already, you will start noticing single-use plastic *everywhere*. It will shock you and, I believe, inspire you to take charge of doing what you can because you'll understand you *can* take charge. Essentially, I am banking on the fact that you will come up with your own simple action plan for plastics once you see the problem and understand your own consumption patterns.

While I cannot go into your home, I can tell you the ten things we did that drastically reduced our single-use plastic and other waste (beyond water bottles and coffee cups):

1. **We stopped buying packaged fruit and vegetables.** In the zero waste world, this is sometimes called "shopping naked." This means no more frozen vegetables, pre-cut vegetables, bagged lettuce, or oranges in plastic net bags.

We buy only package-free produce and we bring our own reusable cotton produce bags. The only produce that we buy frequently that I did not manage to eliminate was raspberries because Matt loves these and he swears they have medicinal properties for him. If you are able to get to a point where it is "just the raspberries" in your life, that's a cause for celebration.

2. **We stopped buying beverages in plastic bottles.** No more orange juice, lemonade or milk in plastic bottles. Cardboard cartons are recyclable so that is what we use. For milk, we found a wonderful alternative in the D.C. area known as South Mountain Creamery (see box below). The milk comes in returnable glass bottles. I have pooled together with three neighbors and we all place a single order every week, which saves us the $5 delivery fee. We all agree the milk tastes better than what we were buying before and it is not more expensive. Some Whole Foods stores offer milk in glass bottles and allow you to get a deposit back when you return the empty bottle. It is worth looking into what's available near you.

3. **We swore off plastic cling wrap.** There are lots of alternatives. Four of my favorites: a plate to cover a bowl, an empty glass jar, reusable bowl covers (see photos below), and Pyrex storage containers. The first two involve no new purchases; the last two do. I love the bowl

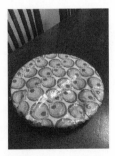 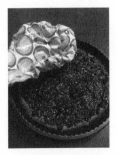

Bowl cover. Photos by Kath Campbell.

Return of the Milkman: Part One

South Mountain Creamery is a family-owned dairy farm in Maryland, which delivers milk in glass bottles weekly to our doorstep. They source from other nearby farms so they are also able to offer a selection of produce and local meat.

I recently asked Tony Brusco, CEO of the company, what his philosophy is about sustainable packaging: "The company considers it a priority to move away from single-use plastic packaging. We pay attention to trends and to what our customers are asking for." As an example, this year they moved from a single-use, plastic-lined ice cream container to a cardboard solution. They invested in the machinery to make the container, and in the long run Tony believes this solution will save them money. That's responsiveness.

---

covers, but honestly, I use the Pyrex storage containers most often. They are great for easy viewing of what's in the fridge, helpful in the quest to avoid food waste.

4. **We started buying dried goods in the bulk aisle.** We no longer buy any of the following items in plastic as they are all available in bulk at several nearby stores: rice, beans, nuts, sugar, flour, spices and even olive oil. For a time during the pandemic, bulk sections of stores closed due to fear of potential contamination. I am happy to say that all the stores we relied on for bulk prior to the pandemic are fully operational again. For more on how we shop in bulk, see the box below.

Zero Waste Grocery Shopping

There is no way around it. If you want to reduce the single-use plastic you bring into your home, you need to alter the way you shop. Here's what I do:

Before I head out to the grocery store or farmers' market, I look at my shopping list and figure out how many containers—mostly reusable cotton produce bags—I will need to bring. I always keep my containers in a grocery shopping bag near the door so they are ready to go. If I plan to buy oranges, apples and lettuce, I'll be sure to have three larger size bags. If I'm planning to shop the bulk aisle for rice, rolled oats and almonds, I'll have another three small or medium-size bags handy. If I'm planning to buy cold cuts or sliced cheese at the deli counter, I bring a stainless steel or Pyrex container.

Once I'm in the store's bulk aisles, I note the number of the product after I've filled my bag to share later with the cashier at checkout. For the deli, I ask the clerk to weigh the item on the store's scale, then place the item in my container, then put the price sticker on top of the container. You can politely say, "I'd like half a pound of Swiss. Please place it in this container after you weigh it." I've never been refused this request.

At checkout, I remind the clerk to deduct the tare which is already on the bag. What is the tare? It is simply the weight of the container (in this case the bag). You don't want to be charged for the weight of the bag itself so you need to know how much your bags weigh. You do this by going to customer service before you start shopping and they can weigh the bags for you. You only need to figure this out once...and then note it on the bag for future shopping.

Lastly, once home, I transfer the dried good items to empty glass jars. For the produce, I try to always wash and prep these so they'll be ready to go when I need them. I then throw all the empty produce bags into the laundry.

5. **We no longer use paper towels, paper napkins, or tissues.** All three are usually wrapped in plastic so finding substitutes eliminates this plastic waste stream and eliminates the waste from these paper products themselves (although they are all compostable). And never purchasing these again saves you money.

Instead of paper towels, I created a non-paper towel system (see photo below). This sounds very fancy, but involves three simple items: 24 washcloths, a bin to store the clean ones on the kitchen counter, and a bin to hold the dirty ones under the sink. You could save even more money by making your own washcloths by cutting up old cotton sheets or T-shirts (use pinking shears to avoid fraying).

Instead of paper napkins, we now use cotton cloth napkins gifted to me over many years by friends. I am not sure why I used to bring these out only for guests in the past. Now we use them at every meal, guests or no guests.

It was hard for me to eliminate facial tissues. Blame it on allergies or just years of a habit of grabbing a tissue for quick clean-ups, but I used to have a tissue box in almost every room. Instead, I bought myself a couple dozen good old-fashioned handkerchiefs and I keep them in a container by my bedside. It means we do not have the same convenience as before, but I never have far to go to get one. We still keep a tissue box on hand for guests or for "emergencies," but I think we are using the same box we started with two months ago.

The reusable versions of paper towels, napkins and hankies do not take up much space and we add these to our laundry loads.

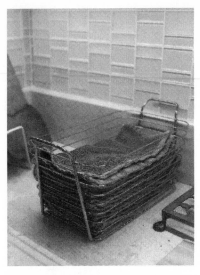

Non-paper towels. Photo by Reyn Anderson.

6. **We bring our own containers for takeout and "doggie bags" for restaurant leftovers.** This may seem challenging at first, but it is hugely rewarding and likely makes you a trend-setter. For takeout, here is what I do: we have a favorite Chinese restaurant that has been in D.C. for decades. I know one of the managers by name; I place my order by phone with Grace and we agree on what time I will drop off my reusable containers. I try to remember to ask for no plastic cutlery or soy sauce packets. About ten minutes after I drop off the containers, the order is packaged and ready. We use this system with a neighborhood Thai restaurant as well. The sacrifice you may need to make: you will need to avoid food delivery since you can't control the containers in that case. And you will need to wait a

few minutes until your food is packaged. That's it. For sit-down meals at restaurants, I always carry a collapsible silicone container with me as a "doggie bag."

7. **We only use a reusable bag at the drycleaners.** As I shared in the introduction, making this simple request at my local cleaners to package our clothes in our own reusable bag launched a different model at that cleaners. A colleague who lives in my neighborhood asked her cleaners to do the same and her cleaner said "no." So she switched to my drycleaners. You will not know the answer until you ask. Nor will the cleaner know her customers have demand for more sustainable packaging until you ask.

8. **We eliminated liquid soap.** This swap was more controversial in our household than I expected. When did we all get so used to liquid soap out of plastic pump bottles? Such a strange addiction. But we are back to bar soap now. Our local farmers' market has a stand that sells unpackaged goats' milk soap and I always place these in my own bag.

9. **We shop at local farmers' markets as much as possible.** These are great sources of "naked produce" — no plastic bags or netting. Plus, the food is always fresh; produce is brought from nearby, minimizing carbon emissions from transport; and you support your local economy. An added benefit: the sense of community as you get to know the salespeople and your fellow shoppers.

10. **We have adopted reusable packaging for shampoo and conditioner.** Any serious zero waste guru will have you make your own shampoo or at least buy shampoo and conditioner sold as bars (they look like soap bars). I tried, but it did not quite do it for my thick hair and Matt and Daniel were immovable on this. The solution: we now buy shampoo and conditioner in reusable metal bottles through Loop, an innovative company that provides

commonly used household products and foods in reusable containers.

Return of the Milkman: Part Two

At the 2019 World Economic Forum, TerraCycle, a company focused on recycling hard-to-recycle items, announced their new venture: partnering with major consumer product groups like Procter & Gamble, Unilever, and PepsiCo, to re-design their packaging to make it reusable. Loop offers these products for delivery through an online platform.

When you finish up, say, your shampoo, you place the bottle into the Loop tote and when your tote is full, UPS, Loop's logistic partner, comes to collect it. Loop then cleans the containers and re-fills them for the next order. I am a regular customer with Loop, and particularly appreciate the laundry detergent, shampoo, Haagen-Dazs ice cream and, lately, disinfecting wipes. For folks who don't have easy access to bulk shopping, they offer a nice array of rice, lentils, nuts and even pasta.

The cost of products offered by Loop is comparable to the cost of the same products you can purchase in stores. The main difference is that there is a delivery fee and you need to pay deposits on the Loop containers, but these are fully refundable. So far, 100,000 people have signed up to be customers, and starting this summer, service will be available to every zip code in the 48 contiguous states in the U.S., as well as in France and the U.K. In 2021, Loop will expand to Canada, Australia and Japan. They also expect to have their products on offer in stores across the U.S. in 2021.

Do consumers have a voice in demanding sustainable

packaging? According to Loop CEO, Tom Szaky, the answer is: "Absolutely. Consumers vote with their pocketbooks. So, as consumers make purchase choices based on sustainability (which is happening now), consumer products companies will have to become more sustainable or their business will suffer. Consumers will be the driving force of change."

Will any one of these actions on their own save the oceans? No. But as you start paying attention to your plastic consumption, you rethink the importance of convenience and start thinking outside the "traditional consumer" box.

Things That Can Derail You

The pandemic. The coronavirus brought a new challenge to the plastics problem: a resurgence in single-use plastic due to health concerns. As we scrambled to find ways to de-contaminate our groceries and avoid touching any surface that someone else may have touched right before us, grocers and coffee shops banned reusables. Safety first. We all had to adjust.

Those of us who had been shopping in bulk aisles to avoid the packaging could no longer bring in our own containers, let alone enter some of the stores with the best bulk buying opportunities. Starbucks and other coffee shops stopped accepting customers' own cups. Lauren Singer, one of the most popular zero waste bloggers, posted a picture of herself looking glum. It was as though all the difficult choices we zero wasters had made so painstakingly were thrown out the window. Our own household became flooded with plastic bags and cardboard boxes from grocery deliveries. Most of us pursuing a low-waste lifestyle felt highly compromised. And a bit depressed.

Three months later, more than 100 health experts across the

globe—epidemiologists, immunologists, and other medical professionals—signed a statement assuring the public that reusables are safe during COVID-19. The statement from scientists came in response to concern that environmental efforts to reduce single-use plastic waste were losing ground due to fears of virus contamination as well as concerns that the plastics industry was exploiting the crisis to lobby against bans on single-use plastics.[7]

This was an important moment of reassurance, and a rebuke of the plastics industry's claim that single-use packaging was safer than reusables. "I hope we can come out of the COVID-19 crisis more determined than ever to solve the pernicious problems associated with plastics in the environment," stated Charlotte K. Williams, a professor of chemistry at Oxford University and one of the signatories of the statement. At the time of this writing, many of the bans on reusables are still in place, but consumers are signing petitions to demand their reversal.

Eating out. Before the pandemic, we ate out several times a month. In nice establishments, avoiding plastic was fairly easy and, if we took leftovers home, I could use my silicone container as described above to avoid any plastic. But what happens when you meet a friend or colleague for lunch at, say, Cava? In an establishment that cares about sustainable packaging (like Cava) you end up with single-use compostable or biodegradable plates and cutlery; but you need to dispose of them properly (see Chapter 4). Many of the less responsible establishments or non-chain establishments that cannot afford the more sustainable packaging will serve your meal in plastic or Styrofoam containers. What can you do? Here is another one of those tough-but-not-as-tough-as-choosing-not-to-fly decisions: you avoid these establishments. I know, not fair. But as my mother always says, life isn't fair.

If you do end up eating somewhere with no reusable options, there is one thing you can do: you can carry a set of reusable

cutlery with you. I carry a bamboo set with me at all times...
I may get some curious, but never hostile looks, from my
lunchmates or other patrons.

* * *

Now that we have discussed all the ways to avoid single-use
plastic, we will next look at what to do when you simply can't
avoid it or other packaging.

Chapter 4

Recycle Right

The human race is challenged more than ever before to demonstrate our mastery, not over nature but of ourselves.
Rachel Carson

Two years ago, the world got a wake-up call about its recycling habits.

In January 2018, China launched its "National Sword" policy, banning the import of plastics and other materials that were being sent to China's recycling processors. Almost overnight the world scrambled to figure out what to do with its waste. Up to that point, 95 percent of European Union and 70 percent of U.S. plastics collected for recycling were sold to Chinese processors.[1]

China wanted to address its own environmental challenges by limiting the level of contamination of materials destined for recycling. Contamination is what happens when trash gets mixed in with recyclables and makes otherwise recyclable items unrecyclable.

China's new policy exposed how reliant the U.S. recycling sector had become on the relationship with China. It turns out there are lots of problems with the U.S. recycling system, and many of these pertain to the global system as well (see box below). Just consider:

- *Only about 50% of Americans have access to curbside recycling*[2]
- *The U.S. recycling rate for plastics is 8 percent and is falling*[3]
- *Of the 367 recycling facilities in the U.S., only 11 percent of them can recycle plastic cups.*[4] Think of that next time

you order at Starbucks as their cups are lined with plastic.

- *The U.S. contamination rate hovers at around 25 to 30 percent*[5] (read: we are lousy recyclers).

Recycling Challenges in the U.S.

There are many issues with recycling in the U.S., but here are the most challenging ones:[6]

Supply. For the benefits of recycling to be realized, more of the recyclable materials we use needs to end up in recycling bins. Currently, only about half of Americans have access to curbside recycling. To make matters worse, curbside recycling has been suspended in many communities during the pandemic while residential waste has increased by up to 35 percent.

Demand. For a market to thrive, there must be demand for products made with recycled content. Consumers can support companies that use recycled materials by buying products labeled "made from recycled content" and by urging companies to offer more such products.

Need for producer incentives. Recycling incentives are needed to hold manufacturers responsible for managing the end-life of their products. This has led to a movement called extended producer responsibility which is not widely implemented due to strong pushback from industry trade groups. There is one success story worth noting: lead batteries, which are recycled at a rate of 99.3 percent, thanks to the combined action by the federal government (passage of the National Battery Act) and states (with many states requiring producers to offer or fund battery recycling).

Inadequate infrastructure. The U.S. recycling system is outdated, and more sophisticated machinery and systems

---

are needed to better sort and process materials. Funding poses a challenge, but manufacturers and the federal government are potential sources.

Misleading labeling Recycling labels on products are confusing, inconsistent and often misleading, as you'll see at the end of this chapter. If the Break Free From Plastic Pollution Act passes, we may finally see standardized labeling for recycling introduced on a national scale.

It would be easy to throw up your hands and give up on recycling until these problems are fixed by governments and industries. But, let's face it, we as consumers are partly to blame as we have been trained that sorting recyclables is a solution to pollution. When it goes in the blue bin, we believe our duty as good environmental citizens is done. As shown in the contamination statistic above, this assumption is harmful.

What made me realize how important it is to recycle right? Good data, of course. The scientists at *Project Drawdown* show that if household recycling rates improved such that the "laggards" (countries and cities whose recycling rates are at 35 percent or lower) increased their recycling rates to the level of the front-runners (with recycling rates of 65 percent or more), 2.8 gigatons of carbon dioxide emissions could be avoided annually by 2050. This is equivalent to taking 600 million cars off the road. We know these increased recycling rates are achievable because they are already being achieved by front-runners across the globe: San Francisco, California; Adelaide, Australia; Quezon City, Philippines; and Bamako, Mali; to name a few.[7]

What can you do?

First you can recycle *less* by finding package-free substitutes for some of the recyclable items as the goal should be to minimize waste in the first place. But as long as packaged products are part of our lifestyle choices, we must get the recycling part right.

Consider touring your local Materials Recycling Facility (MRF, rhymes with "Smurf"). This is the next stop (not the last stop) for everything you put in your recycling bin. It is where everything is sorted by material and packaged into bales (see photo below), which are then purchased by off-takers who do the actual recycling of the material. I do not consider touring a recycling facility to be an 80/20 action because it does take time to do. But it is eye-opening and worthwhile.

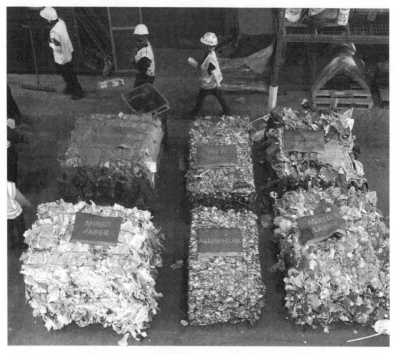

**Prince George's County, Maryland Materials Recycling Facility.
Photo by Stephanie Miller.**

I have toured all the recycling facilities in my region open to the public (call me a recycling nerd) and I am in regular contact with recycling experts. I email my local recycling representative several times a month to ask whether this or that is accepted for recycling and I always get a thoughtful answer. It's great to get it 100 percent right, but you don't need to.

You do, however, need to let go of "wish-cycling," that tendency we all have of throwing something into the recycling bin in the hopes that it is recyclable. Recycling right helps ensure efficiency and the profitability of the recycling system (think about your tax dollars). It can also ensure greater worker safety at the sorting facilities.

And in case you need another reason, in some jurisdictions, like Washington, D.C., improper recycling can result in a fine. Right before the pandemic, the D.C. office that handles waste sent around postcards about a $75 fine that would be imposed for poor recycling practices.

You have no doubt heard the expression "What gets measured, gets done." In the business world I was a part of for more than two decades, accountability for performance measures was key to seeing results. When my group started tracking our climate investments and we were able to get "percentage of climate-smart business" on our institution's "scorecard" for tracking results, we saw a 50 percent jump in business in less than three years following a decade of stagnation.

Measuring your recycling trash today—knowing your starting point—will arm you with the information you need to waste less and recycle better. Enter the audit. Put on your gloves and I'll walk you through this.

The 80/20 Recycling Plan
Recycle Right Action Step: Conduct a Recycle Bin Audit

An audit sounds like a big, important and boring process. Something you hire an accountant to do for you. This audit is very simple. As with all audits, it involves two things: data collection and analysis.

Know your trash... aka data collection. Let's break this down into four simple steps:

1. Prepare the week before: Decide on the date you will do the audit. It should ideally be the day before your recycling pick-up day. If your municipality does single-stream collection (all recycling placed in one container), then separate glass items in another bag or bin for the week leading up to the audit to avoid glass breakage when you pour everything out of the bin for the audit.

2. On the day of your audit, pick a flat surface, spread out a tarp or a towel and separate your recycling items into four piles according to what they are made of: 1) plastic 2) metal 3) glass and 4) cardboard and paper.

3. Take some pictures of the items while they are spread out. Take one picture of the whole scene with all the piles, and then take one close-up of each of the four piles.

4. Sort for recyclability, ensuring you have not included anything that does not belong there. How do you do that? Check your local guidelines to be sure that everything you are putting in your recycling bin is accepted. You can usually find your local guidelines by googling "recycling rules near me." Here are the ten most common mistakes people make:

   • **Plastic bags.** Do not place these in your municipal recycling bin. I confess: a few years ago, I used to bag my recycling items in plastic grocery bags before placing them in the bin. Here's the problem with that: if these bags are not successfully sifted out by the sorters at the very first stage of the process, they can get caught in the sorting machinery and shut down the entire plant for several hours. In fact, at MRFs across the U.S., this happens several times a day. Often the workers at the facility need to use box cutters to cut out the plastic, a tricky process that can lead to worker injury.

When I asked representatives of my local MRFs about their number one challenge, the answer has been consistently: "Plastic bags are 90 percent of the problem." Please gently tell everyone you know to keep plastic bags out of the recycling bins and instead take them to grocery stores for collection by participating partners. See Appendix 1 for Grocery Store Recycling Cheat Sheet.

- **Dirty containers.** You will need to rinse and dry your containers before placing them in your recycling bin to avoid contaminating other items in your bin. You do not need to scrub but you need to get most of the food or drink off by rinsing them out. I usually leave these in the dry rack overnight before putting them in the bin the next day.
- **Pizza boxes.** As an example of the last point, oil cannot easily be separated from the paper fiber of pizza boxes. So here's what you can do: the top part of the pizza box is almost always fairly food free. If this is the case, tear off the top from the bottom and place the mostly food-free top into the recycling bin. If the bottom part is greasy, it should go in the trash or in your compost bin, if you have one.
- **Textiles/Clothing.** These are often mistakenly placed in recycling bins, but they are not accepted by municipal MRFs. There are lots of options for disposal of clothing. They can be donated or swapped, if they are in good condition. If stained or torn, they *can* be recycled at certain locations (google Earth911's Recycling Locator) and some companies accept their clothing back. I like to donate old sheets to animal shelters, which are always in need, and lately, I have cut up cotton textiles to make into reusable non-paper towels.

- **Batteries.** These are considered hazardous waste because they are made of metals which are harmful to humans and animals. They should not be placed in your regular recycling bin. Some municipalities allow you to place *some* batteries in your regular trash. Check your local guidelines for special drop-off points for batteries and electronics.
- **Shredded paper.** This was a surprise to me. I had always proudly bagged my shredded paper and placed it in the recycling bin. Paper is recyclable but shredded paper is usually not welcome in your curbside bin. Why not? The answer is that the fibers are too short to work well in the machines. A great solution for shredded paper is to use it in your compost bin; it serves as the "brown" (think dried leaves) that mixes so well with the vegetable scraps. If you do not compost or use a compost service, you can save shredded paper for wrapping delicate items you might ship. But who ships that much delicate stuff? As with so many other things, when you realize there is no great end-of-life place for something, you start to think of how you can reduce it. Maybe you do not need to shred everything that comes through in the mail? Just the really sensitive information? Check your municipality for special drop-off points for shredded paper.
- **Plastic wrap.** This was another surprise to me and almost everyone I know. It is plastic, so it should be recyclable, right? Well, not all plastic is created equal and not all of it is acceptable for recycling. Plastic film (think thin plastic such as grocery bags, packaging around toilet paper and paper towels, plastic bread bags) belongs in one of two places: 1) the grocery store for take-back programs offered by participating partners or 2) the trash (see plastics section below).

- **Black plastic.** These are the containers many restaurants use for takeout orders. The top is often clear (and usually recyclable), but the bottom is often black (and not recyclable). Who knew? I did not until recently. Even though you'll often see the little triangle (perhaps with the number "5" inside) that would lead you to believe this can be placed in your recycling bin, it turns out that almost no facilities are able to properly sort these. This is because of an obscure sorting issue: the facilities use an infrared optical sorter which cannot detect the plastic item if it is black.
- **Paper napkins and towels.** You can compost these, but they should not be placed in your curbside recycling bin. If you do not compost, place these in the trash.
- **Items smaller than 2 by 2 inches.** These should not be placed in your curbside recycling because they will slip through the cracks of the sorting machinery at the recycling plant. This can be very confusing because many small plastic items—like aspirin containers, lip gloss pots, plastic cutlery—do have a recycling symbol with a number inside indicating what plastic they are made of (the "resin identification code"). But their small size trumps their material when it comes to recyclability.

Now that you have sifted out everything that *does not* belong in your recycling bin, you are done for the day. Place all the recyclable items back in the recycling bin. That's it... you've collected all your data and completed the first part.

Analyze your trash. You now have the data you need to evaluate your household's recycling habits. You want to look for opportunities to reduce your waste. Let's go back to the waste hierarchy: reduce, reuse, recycle. Your goal in reducing waste is to first reduce your consumption of items that are packaged.

Is there anything you think you could easily eliminate? Every person/household is different, but here are some examples of what you might consider:

You notice in the plastics or the glass pile that you have a large quantity of empty carbonated water bottles. Perhaps sparkling water is not something you are willing to give up, but you might conclude that it would be worthwhile investing in a carbonator, such as SodaStream. Buying one—new or, even better, used— would save on all those disposable bottles.

You notice a lot of plastic yogurt containers. You could try your hand at making your own yogurt, as my friend Reyn decided to do once she found herself with some extra time during the pandemic. Or you could try buying your yogurt in larger containers to save on the plastic.

As I did in the last chapter, I am recommending the audit as your *one action step* for recycling because I believe every household is different and you can easily devise your own plan once the audit reveals where the opportunities lie.

The Piles. Now let's look at each pile in order, starting with plastics.

Plastics. Your goal should be to get this pile as small as possible. Chapter 2 should help you navigate alternatives. I suggest you do another audit in, say, six months, and aim to shrink this plastics pile substantially. Beyond the common mistakes listed above, let's really nail this to be sure your plastics are in the right place.

You can discard used plastics in one of three places:

- your residential recycling bin
- designated collection bins at your grocery store, or
- your trash can

Here are the steps to take to know which of the three options is right. It may seem tedious, but once you start doing this regularly, you will not have to think about it. I promise.

Step 1: Ask yourself: Is the plastic item solid like a plastic bottle or flimsy like a plastic bag? If solid, go to Step 2. If flimsy, skip to Step 3.

Step 2: For solid plastics, what is the number inside the resin identification code, the triangular symbol? If there is no number, it is probably not recyclable. Frown and toss it in the trash can.

If there is a number, use the cheat sheet offered in Appendix 1, which you can even tape alongside your municipal recycling rules on your fridge or near your recycling bin as handy reminders. *It is really important to note that the codes were created as a communications tool for manufacturers. They were not intended for consumers.* But until a better system is developed, we need some guidance to help us navigate the tangled web of plastics recycling decisions.

Step 3: Flimsy bags and other "plastic film" packaging labeled with a "2" or a "4" in the triangle should go to your grocery store drop-off point. Often, there is no number at all on these items. A good test is to check whether the plastic is stretchy or crinkly. The stretchy stuff is usually accepted; the crinkly is usually not.

What happens to the plastic you drop off at the grocery store? Participating grocery stores partner with private companies, such as Trex, which in turn recycle the plastic into items such as deck furniture and flooring. In my area, participating grocery stores include: Giant, Safeway, Wegmans and Whole Foods.

Metals. The wonderful thing I learned during my first tour of a materials recycling center is that metals are infinitely recyclable. *Recycled aluminum requires 95 percent less energy to produce than virgin metals,*[7] so there is a large environmental benefit to recycling metals. The other amazing thing I learned is that metals recycling is so efficient that an aluminum can is recycled, repurposed and back on the store shelf in 60 days.

This should provide you with some comfort when you gaze at your metals pile. Cans should be rinsed out to minimize the chance for contamination. The lid can be placed inside the can for safe disposal. You can also recycle foil pans and tin foil. In most jurisdictions, you should create a tin foil ball at least two inches in diameter (aim for baseball size) so that the foil does not fall through the cracks (literally) in the sorting process.

The metals stream is very profitable, so the MRFs rely on this income to cover their expenses.

Glass. This material brings me joy and heartache all at once. The joy comes from the beauty and purity of glass, and from my discovery of so many reuses for glass containers. I had a whole shelf built to accommodate the glass jars that came into my life when I began my zero waste efforts (see photo below). And this picture does not give a sense of all the other jars in our cupboards and freezer. Any serious zero waster will extol the virtues of glass jars. In fact, I would say the glass mason jar became the mascot of the zero waste movement ever since Bea Johnson, the founder of the movement, was famously pictured holding a mason jar of her annual trash. Kathryn Kellogg does this as well in her book *101 Ways to Go Zero Waste*. It is good to have lofty goals.

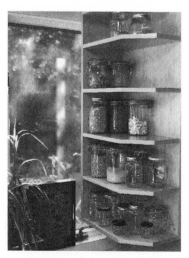

Photo by Stephanie Miller.

Like metals, glass is infinitely recyclable and using cullet (recycled glass) in the glass manufacturing process saves significant energy compared to processing virgin materials.

The heartache came from learning that there are big problems with recycling glass in the U.S. Unlike in Europe, where glass recycling rates average 73 percent, the U.S. rate is only 34 percent.[9] There are many reasons for this. One reason in the U.S. (but not in Europe) is that the distances from MRFs to glass manufacturers can be prohibitively far and transportation costs of glass are very high because the material is heavy.

Another problem is that most of the U.S. uses a single-stream collection which, on the one hand, makes it easier for households to throw recyclables in one place. On the other hand, broken glass gets into the other recycling streams and can render these streams less valuable. This is one of the reasons that Arlington County, Virginia made the decision in 2019 to no longer accept glass in its recycling bin. Instead, the county has installed separate glass collection points and the glass is used as aggregate for road paving, construction and landscaping. I was dismayed to learn this about Arlington County until I learned that in D.C. glass is collected, but diverted to the landfill rather than recycled. I've been told that D.C. has not given up on the prospect of recycling glass but for now using it as landfill cover is the most economical solution.

What does this mean for you? It means that you should find out whether your municipality does, in fact, recycle glass. If it does, then you should favor this material in your packaging. If it does not, then you might consider alternatives. For example, I have been advising people in my vicinity to consider beer in cans rather than glass bottles. Even better, of course, is to buy beer in reusable glass growlers.

Paper and Cardboard. These can both be recycled, but not infinitely like metals and glass. The paper fibers break down each time they undergo the recycling process until they are no longer usable... about 5–7 times. Still, it is important to recycle them. When we recycle cardboard and paper, we save precious resources and energy: recycling one ton of paper saves 17 trees and 7000 gallons of water.[10] The figures for cardboard savings are even greater.

Check your municipality's rules on paper recycling, including whether they accept shredded paper and whether you should break down your cardboard boxes.

If you find yourself with large piles of cardboard boxes in your recycling bin, there are ways to reduce, of course. Are the boxes the result of a lot of Amazon or other deliveries? If so, you might ask: do you really need all the stuff you are ordering? Would you consider trying a month of buying nothing new? Or consider waiting a week before any impulse purchases and see if you really need the item. You might also want to explore the *sharing economy* concept (more on this in the next chapter).

If you find yourself with large piles of paper, perhaps it is unwanted mail? If so, the painstaking process of contacting each of the senders pays off as you see your junk mail practically vanish. Less painstaking is to use mail-preference services like DMAchoice.org to opt out of direct mail and CatalogChoice.org to cancel catalogs. It takes less than five minutes to log on to DMAchoice and the service will cancel your direct mail for ten years at a charge of $2. Catalog Choice is a free service that lets you cancel specific catalogs. This will not put a stop to all junk mail but you will notice a big difference. Of course, I would strongly suggest that you do as much as possible of your bill paying and banking online.

Handy Tips

Make recycling right easier for everyone. Perhaps you buy into all the benefits of recycling and you are already an avid recycler yourself, but your housemates may not share your passion. Some advice:

First, make it easier for everyone in your household by having clearly marked bins for each purpose.

Second, be gentle. You might feel frustrated as you remind your partner for the third time that the black plastic takeout container needs to go in the trash, not the recycling bin. Admit to yourself that you are the household recycling expert, give yourself a pat on the back, move the container to the correct bin, and consider giving a fourth reminder. Be extra appreciative the next time your partner gets it right.

Beware of greenwashing. I think I could write a whole book on the suffix "*-able.*" Compost*able*, Biodegrad*able*, Recycl*able*. With consumers more eager for green alternatives to packaging, companies are more eager than ever to please. And this can lead to marketing ploys and greenwashing, unsubstantiated claims about how environmentally-friendly a company or its products are. It can also lead to a lot of confusion.

What does it mean to be "recyclable"? It means *able* to be recycled. But by whom? And where? If four billion Starbucks coffee cups per year are technically recyclable, but only 11 percent of recycling facilities in the U.S. have the equipment *able* to recycle them, then we are "wish-cycling" when we place our non-reusable coffee cup in the recycling bin at Starbucks.

Ok, so what about "compost*able*? And what is the difference between biodegradable and compostable. According to Earth911: "Compostable and biodegradable are often used interchangeably. But they are not the same thing. Biodegradable means that a product can be broken down *without* oxygen and that it turns into carbon dioxide, water and biomass within a reasonable amount of time."[11] A compostable item is assumed to use oxygen in the decomposition process.

Now, let me give you an example of why the concept of compostable packaging is tricky. We have two dogs. Dog poop bags are a dilemma. Is it better to use a plastic newspaper sleeve or a compostable dog poop bag? The answer may surprise you.

If you use a compostable bag, but you put your poop-filled bag into the trash, then you are not allowing the bag to compost. The composting process only happens when specific levels of heat, water and oxygen are achieved. These conditions are not present in the landfill. They are most likely not even present in home composting systems, which don't normally reach the heat levels required to compost dog poop bags (not to mention that you shouldn't place your dog's poop in your home composting pile for sanitary reasons as it contains bacteria and possibly parasites). So, you are not doing anything better for the environment when you purchase compostable poop bags that end up in the landfill. If you are still receiving paper newspapers at your doorstep, the best thing you can do is to reuse the plastic sleeves they come in for your dog walks rather than buy new dog bags, whether labeled as compostable or not.

Creating more sustainable packaging is a worthwhile endeavor. But, for sustainable packaging to work, it needs to be supported by proper labeling collection practices, accessible technology and consumer education. We still have a long way to go to get there.

Chapter 5

Beyond the Individual

There comes a time when humanity is called to shift to a new level of consciousness . . . that time is now.
Wangari Maathai

The Unexpected Joys of Going Zero Waste

A few years ago, I packed up and left Paris, France, where I had been posted as the head of IFC's Western Europe group. Though eager to return to my D.C. home and friends after three years abroad, I was also keenly aware of what I would miss about Paris. When you live in Paris, you don't actually live in Paris; you live in your *quartier* in Paris, your immediate neighborhood. In three short years, I got to know more people by name in my *quartier*—shopkeepers at our local bakery, hair salon, butcher shop, and the florist around the corner—than I ever knew after decades in my D.C. neighborhood. In saying goodbye to Paris, I also left behind the warmth of my newfound community.

Little did I know that going zero waste would re-create this kind of community back in D.C. Remember my story of the reusable bags at the drycleaners? How unlikely that would have been without my long-standing relationship with the owner. To avoid plastic containers for takeout at my favorite Chinese restaurant, I got to know Grace by name—she is almost always the one taking phone orders and now knows that I will bring my own containers. Same thing with Sue, Bob and Walter at the local fish market—one quick call and they leave my seafood ready and unpackaged on ice until I arrive. At our weekly farmers' market, it is a pleasure to greet Pallavi, Brett, Alfredo and Kim. If I want to order Kim's delicious apple cake but avoid the single-use plastic clamshell, I drop off my container one week, and the next Kim has it ready with my treat. At our local grocer, Broad Branch Market, Tracy and John, Ana and Mihret let me shop with my own jars or bags for bulk items and produce... no questions asked. These relationships make sustainable shopping easier, while building a sense of community. It is a great feeling.

Another unexpected joy: learning how to do more on my own, feeling resourceful and self-sufficient. I went from happily paying a service to pick up our compost scraps every week to eventually relishing my own backyard composting. How satisfying when I dump the kitchen bucket into our composting bin, knowing that I am diverting all this waste from the landfill and with it, needless methane emissions.

I have also picked up gardening. With Matt, who is luckily more experienced in the garden than I am, we went from seedlings to a bountiful harvest of tomatoes, peppers, and herbs. There is something special about eating delicious home-grown tomatoes.

Last summer my multi-talented uncle, Steve, taught me how to sew so that I could make my own cloth produce bags from old sheets. Now I can sew fairly straight lines and do what it takes to make produce bags for myself and my friends.

And then there is clothes shopping. I have never enjoyed clothes shopping, not in stores or online, but I am told shopping in thrift stores is becoming trendy. What great news from a zero waste perspective. Thrifting offers a counterpoint to "fast fashion" — cheap, trendy clothing that generates 11 million tons of textile waste per year in the U.S. alone.[1] And that's not all: the fashion industry contributes about ten percent of annual global greenhouse gas emissions, and toxic chemicals used in the dyeing process pollute water systems.[2] Since I'm not the best advocate for any clothes shopping, I asked Torin O'Brien, an avid "thrifter" I know, to describe the allure (see box below).

Thrills of Thrifting

Here is how Torin O'Brien, an 18-year-old living in Washington, D.C., describes the appeal of thrifting:

Finding something at a thrift store means that it is one of a kind. For those of us who use clothes to distinguish ourselves, a unique item is one of the best ways to do so. I love that the clothes at thrift stores come from a wide variety of people and time periods. A bright orange tank top or ankle length skirt in a thrift shop invites creativity in my closet. Inexpensive secondhand clothing also gives me and my friends the freedom to explore our sense of style while still staying within our weekly allowance.

Thrifting clothes gives me the freedom to alter them without guilt. When an item is low cost, the idea of tailoring or embroidering it is less daunting. I initially learned how to sew so I could alter a skirt I'd thrifted and which didn't quite fit. I feel less restricted working on found pieces of clothing because my mistakes won't cost them the entirety of their usefulness. After changing a piece to fit me perfectly, whether by taking something in or sewing in tiny embroidered flowers, I am less likely to throw it away.

Thrifting, ultimately, creates connections between people and their surroundings. It helps me feel closer to my community when I shop at these small, often non-profit stores. I love that it helps me have a positive impact on the world by saving clothes from waste and giving them a new life.

The Ripple Effect

Let's return to the three questions I asked myself as I started looking at ways to reduce my waste and carbon footprint.

1. What can we—as individuals—do to reverse the current climate and waste crises?
2. Could individual actions have a ripple effect that could lead to systemic change?
3. If so, how could busy people contribute to making these systemic changes?

I hope I have answered the first question throughout the book... we, as individuals, can do a lot.

So now let us look at the second and third questions. An individual's efforts can make a difference if the changes they make inspire others to do the same. We have all seen what happened with the plastic straw after Milo Cress, the 9-year-old Vermont boy, started a movement to ban them: in a relatively short period, they have become practically taboo. Or think of the face mask: do you know anyone who was wearing one in January 2020? Now, people in most communities around the globe wear them because they understand doing so matters.

If you adopt a plant-based diet, reduce your food waste, compost, seek more sustainable packaging, and recycle with care, you can inspire others to do the same.

Where can your precious time make the most difference? Should you focus on your friends and colleagues? Or is your time better spent emailing the businesses you patronize to let them know your preferences? Or are you likely to be most effective by writing to your local politician? The answer is: it depends. Below are ideas on how to extend your reach as a member of your community, as a consumer and as a constituent.

Influencing Your Community

How much can your individual actions influence those around you? I recently put this question to Diogo Veríssimo, a Research Fellow at the University of Oxford who applies social marketing theory and tools to address conservation challenges. He says that what we learn from the plastic straw example is that change can happen quickly and it does not need to take generations.

The key is understanding the power of individual behavior to set social norms. Don't underestimate the important signal you send to your peers when, say, at the end of a meal you ask where you can place your recyclables. By doing so, you are sending the message about your expectation that recycling should be available. In other words, what your peers *think* is the right thing to do does *matter*.

Veríssimo cites a well-known study on the power of social norms conducted more than a decade ago by Dr. Robert Cialdini, an Arizona State University professor who spent his career researching the psychology of influence. The study looked at what it takes to get hotel guests to choose to reuse their towels during their hotel stay. It turns out that when guests found a sign in their bathroom not only telling them about the environmental benefits of reusing their towels, but also letting them know that a majority of hotel guests reuse their towels, they were 26 percent more likely to opt for reusing their towels compared to guests who only saw a sign about the environmental benefits.[3]

The interesting thing about modeling behavior is that, for it to be effective, the model needs to be someone you identify with. Here is where *you* come in. There is no one else in the world who has access to your social circles other than you. And Veríssimo believes that, especially in the age of social media, we can showcase our pro-environmental behavior and push for a change in what is perceived to be the norm.

That is a lot of power for each of you reading this. Imagine if 500 people reading this book model social norms that inspire just ten people each. And if those 5000 people inspire another ten each. That is a ripple effect involving 50,000 people. Not bad for the little time invested in modeling behavior in your community.

What you can do:

Use social media. I was a slow adopter and will certainly never be as savvy on this front as Millennials and Gen Zs. Nonetheless, I have enjoyed getting more proficient on Instagram.

Whether it's sharing a great vegetarian recipe, showing how you used leftovers for a creative meal to avoid food waste, or bringing your own sustainable packaging for takeout or grocery shopping, your connections on social media will take notice of your actions. And you create social norms by sharing your own behaviors.

Cooking on Instagram

A favorite thing I've done in the past year was to create a vegetarian *cookalong*, which I post about on Instagram and Facebook. It makes me feel as though I'm cooking with friends, and I love comparing notes after we've tried the new recipes.

The way it works is simple: once a week, I choose a vegetarian recipe I want to try and we all separately cook the meal in our own homes. Afterwards, I post my review (and hope I remembered to take a picture of the meal before eating it). Whenever possible, I choose recipes that are available online for free.

You might consider doing the same or some variation of this. You could agree with a handful of friends that you will all cook the same meal on the same night. Without proselytizing, you can bring several people along with you in expanding their vegetarian cuisine. And the next time you have friends over for dinner, consider making a great vegetarian dish they'll want to try making themselves. *My philosophy is: Every Meal Counts.*

My only caveat is to avoid the shame game. I am much more effective at convincing people to try something when I am bursting with enthusiasm than when I cite dire statistics about the importance of, say, a plant-rich diet. Leading with positivity is key to success.

Be a collection point. Once you start noticing the reduction in your waste, you will probably start wondering how much your neighbors and friends are wasting. Don't judge; just think how you might help them.

Did you decide that you would return your corks for *upcycling* (the process of turning discarded items into new products, like creating yoga blocks from used cork) to a liquor store that accepts them? If so, text your friends in advance and offer to drop theirs off as well. Did you invest in a TerraCycle box that allows you to send in your empty coffee bags for recycling? Let your friends know so they can drop their empty coffee bags with you and you can add them to your TerraCycle box before sending it for recycling.

Two of my favorite "collection point" examples come from Catherine Plume, who chairs the D.C. Chapter of Sierra Club. When Catherine began composting, she invited her neighbors to drop off their food scraps on her porch and she would compost these as well. That is a generous act, which introduces her neighbors to the idea of composting.

The other thing she did was to create a party box from thrifted cloth napkins, silverware and plates. Her friends and neighbors know she has this party box and when someone is hosting a party they are welcome to borrow it, avoiding the waste that comes from disposables. I just love this.

Create your own *sharing economy*. We might associate the *sharing economy* with Airbnb and Uber. But we can also view it as an opportunity much closer to home. Cambridge Dictionary defines the *sharing economy* as an economic system based on people sharing possessions and services, either for free or for payment.

My friend Kath created a WhatsApp group for six of us friends that we call "Giveaways, needs, loans" (not the most alluring name, I know). We have exchanged everything from the most banal—think flour, lamps and books—to more obscure things like red miso, a labeling machine and an old fridge. If you are trying to reduce your purchases (and your expenses), as well as move away from compulsive Amazon one-click buying, this is a great first and, often, last stop.

Along the same lines, you can find, give away, sell and buy a lot of items through online platforms. Much like thrift shopping for clothes, I used to think secondhand was second best. Now I see it as a great idea for giving new life to an item that would otherwise end up in the landfill. Using platforms like *Trash Nothing, Nextdoor and Craig's List*, I have purchased used bikes and books and given away cardboard boxes, furniture, and a hair straightener.

These sharing economy ideas require a mental shift away from "new is always better" and a willingness to take the extra step to post a picture or a message before doing an Amazon search. These are small steps that take minutes, not hours or days. And sometimes your neighbor's borrowed waffle iron will be at your disposal even before that Amazon package could arrive at your doorstep.

Influencing as a Consumer

As with so many aspects of the individual's actions, your influence as a consumer may feel like a drop in the bucket. But as we heard in Chapter 2 from the CEOs of *Loop* and *South Mountain Creamery*, your purchasing power counts for a lot. Chad Frischmann, Vice President and Research Director at *Project Drawdown*, puts it this way:

The decisions we all make every day, particularly those of

us in high-income countries, about the food we purchase and consume are some of the most important actions we can take to address climate change. Choosing to purchase more plant-based foods locally grown from organic or regenerative practices, packaged using sustainable materials, and in quantities that we can and will actually consume, sends signals across the value chain to businesses – from groceries to distributors, packagers to farmers – who respond by switching more and more to sustainable solutions.

This tells us we should choose wisely the businesses we patronize, the products we buy there, and how they are packaged. What you can do:

Don't be shy. At your local coffee shop or favorite restaurant, there are easy ways you can advocate for more sustainable packaging.

Try this: next time you are in your favorite coffee shop and you are planning to stay and drink your beverage there, ask the salesclerk if you can have your tea or coffee in a ceramic mug. If they have one available (some Starbucks do, some don't, for instance), you are signaling your interest to the establishment about their stocking reusable mugs (and setting a social norm for nearby customers in the process). If they do not have ceramic mugs available, ask if they would consider offering them to customers.

Bonus points if you speak to the manager about this. It can be as simple as: "I love having my coffee here, but I am trying hard to reduce single-use packaging and would be so happy to be able to drink from a reusable mug." You can be a polite squeaky wheel.

At restaurants, be sure to always have your own container available to bring home leftovers. You might be setting a social norm if other restaurant patrons catch a glimpse of you in action.

Use your consumer dollars to support businesses doing the

right thing. Choose locally-sourced foods as much as possible (e.g., your farmers' market) and look for zero waste stores or at least stores with a selection of items sold in bulk. To find them, google "zero waste store (or bulk store) near me," or search on one of these two platforms for bulk stores: *Litterless' Where to Grocery Shop*, which tracks bulk stores by state in the U.S.; or *Zero Waste Home's Bulk Finder*, which tracks them in the U.S. and Canada.

On the subject of Canada, Tina Soldovieri, a woman living in a neighborhood of Toronto known as Roncesvalles (aka Roncy), teamed up with neighbors to visit local businesses to get them to offer customers the option of bringing their own bags and containers. A total of 73 stores — grocers, bulk food stores, take-out restaurants and even clothing stores — agreed. Each one put a sticker in the window indicating it was part of the *Roncy Reduces* initiative. The concept took off and is now being replicated in 20 other neighborhoods and towns in and outside of Toronto. If I lived in Roncesvalles, I would patronize these stores for all my needs.

And what about supporting a *reuse* company? Remember recycling comes after *reduce* and *reuse* because recycling takes energy. I was thrilled to learn about a local company called Plastic Tree trying to solve this problem and I am now a customer of theirs (see box below).

Reuse, Reuse, Reuse

Plastic Tree is a D.C.-based start-up founded in 2019 which offers an innovative way to make the concept of *reuse* more accessible. Plastic Tree's founder, Lara Ilao, realized many of us want to do the right thing — like return our glass milk bottles for deposits or figure out what to do with bubble wrap or once-used plastic takeout containers — but we simply don't have time.

Plastic Tree helps solve this problem by providing a relatively inexpensive ($8/week) waste management pick-up service: customers place their reusable items into a 20-pound bin and Plastic Tree finds a new home for them. With their six-month pilot now complete, the company found the items they collected fall into two categories: 1) those that can be repaired and then re-sold or donated (e.g. a keyboard missing one key), and 2) durable items that can be reused, such as cardboard boxes and Styrofoam coolers (e.g. the kind often used to transport food or medication). For this second category, Plastic Tree is engaging with businesses (local end markets) to offer these for reuse. For example, Lara is in contact with local breweries to sell them empty beer bottles. Great concept, don't you think?

Influencing as a Constituent

Your vote matters, and so does your voice as a constituent. D.C. Councilmember Mary Cheh who is an environmentalist and a zero waste advocate in her own right, recently shared with me her thoughts on how we, as busy individuals, can be most effective in influencing our politicians on environmental issues.

Our environmental output is the culmination of everyone's individual decisions, so my first recommendation to anyone looking to make a difference would be to incorporate new sustainability measures within his or her own life. And when those changes are implemented, share how they have improved your daily experience, health, finances, home, etc. Lead by example and be a vocal and enthusiastic cheerleader for personal change among neighbors, family, and friends.

Obviously, I couldn't agree more. Councilmember Cheh goes on to say:

> And for those environmental efforts that can only be met at the broader policy level, the best way the average person can advocate for these critical environmental causes is to make it personal. You may be asked by a local or national organization to sign a petition or send a form letter to an elected official, but, at the end of the day, your personal story and your words are what matter most. Customize that form letter to demonstrate how action is needed now and how this issue, whatever it may be, affects your daily life. Let your representative know why this issue must be a priority above all the others competing for his or her time and political capital. And, whenever you're able, join those community meetings or public forums where the representative will be in attendance and make your case in person.

Your voice as a constituent can make a difference in pushing for better regulation around food waste, composting, plastics and recycling. Here are some things you can do in these areas:

Advocate for less food waste and more composting. Waste collection is a local issue. Imagine if composting were offered as a curbside pick-up service along with your trash and recycling? This happens all over Canada and much of Europe, yet only in rare cases in the U.S., but that doesn't mean we shouldn't ask for it. Consider writing or calling your local councilmember and asking the simple question: "When can I expect curbside composting to be offered in [fill-in-the-blank city]?"

There is growing awareness about food waste and its strong link to climate change and it's heartening to know that a growing number of states are taking action to restrict food waste going to landfills: currently, California, Connecticut, Massachusetts, Rhode Island and Vermont. Find out if your state has progressive legislation pending and then weigh in with a short email or call.

Advocate for less plastics and more and better recycling. Plastics and recycling are inter-related issues which need to be tackled by governments at every level. In the U.S., Congress introduced a bill known as the Break Free from Plastic Pollution Act in February 2020. It includes measures to ensure extended producer responsibility (the concept that manufacturers are held accountable for properly disposing of consumer product packaging), develop standardized recycling and composting labels for products and receptacles, and control plastic factory pollutants.

At the federal and state levels, look for ways to support legislation that seeks to increase recycling rates and provide better consumer education on local recycling rules and bans or puts taxes on single-use plastics. Use govtrak.us/congress/members to find out who your representatives are. This site is also helpful in tracking pending environmental legislation and to know whom to write or call about it.

The Choice

We have entered the decade of reckoning when it comes to climate change. According to climate scientists, we have about nine years to change the current greenhouse gas emissions trajectory. That's nine years to get global temperatures to levels that will avoid the most catastrophic effects of global warming. According to a statement by the U.N. Secretary-General, Antonio Guterres, "The year 2020 will be pivotal for climate action if the world is to control ever worsening impacts and indicators of climate change before it is too late."[4]

As complex as climate change seems and as difficult as reducing waste can be, we have a really simple choice: take action or throw in the towel. That's it. Two choices.

I hope I have convinced you that you can reduce your carbon footprint and waste, inspire others, and influence businesses and government, all while keeping your day job.

When you consciously choose to make a change, you become the kind of person who creates change. You develop agency, and you become more aware of your power and its possibilities to engender changes you believe in. By embracing zero waste, you can become part of a movement towards meaningful action to reverse both climate change and the waste crisis.

Have I managed to take the action steps I have recommended 100 percent of the time? The honest answer is, no. But I do them at least 80 percent of the time. Some weeks we are too tired to plan meals and end up burdened with the inevitable food waste and takeout containers, but we are back on track the following week. As with any behavioral change, it takes some time to get it right. The first step is the hardest: the decision to act.

Epilogue

This morning I woke up to put the finishing touches on the last chapter. Matt poured me some coffee as he hurried to have his breakfast. "Have I mentioned to you how much I love this homemade granola? Would you mind making some more tomorrow since we're almost out." Hope is in the air.

Appendix 1: Cheat Sheets

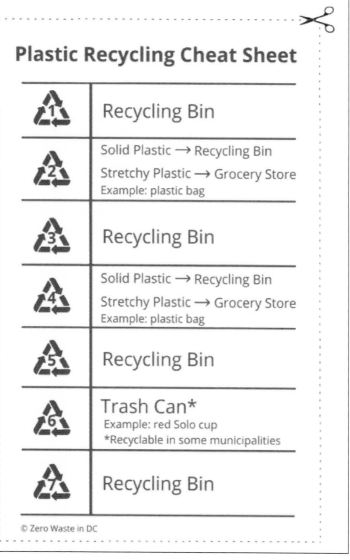

Plastic Recycling Cheat Sheet

△ 1	Recycling Bin
△ 2	Solid Plastic → Recycling Bin Stretchy Plastic → Grocery Store Example: plastic bag
△ 3	Recycling Bin
△ 4	Solid Plastic → Recycling Bin Stretchy Plastic → Grocery Store Example: plastic bag
△ 5	Recycling Bin
△ 6	Trash Can* Example: red Solo cup *Recyclable in some municipalities
△ 7	Recycling Bin

© Zero Waste in DC

Courtesy of Victoria Mills

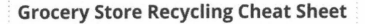

Grocery Store Recycling Cheat Sheet

The following are accepted by participating grocery stores:

- Grocery bags
- Bread bags
- Dry cleaning bags
- Newspaper sleeves
- Ziploc food storage bags
- Cereal bags

Here are common items that should not be placed in curbside recycling bins or dropped off at grocery stores:

- Degradable/compostable bags
- Pre-washed salad mix bags
- Frozen food bags
- Candy bar wrappers
- Chip bags
- Saran wrap

© Zero Waste in DC

Courtesy of Victoria Mills

Appendix 2: Favorite Recipes

Homemade Granola
Recipe adapted from TinyTrashCan.com

Ingredients

3 cups rolled oats
1 ¼ cups sliced almonds or chopped walnuts
½ cup sunflower seeds
1 tablespoon hemp hearts
1 tablespoon wheat germ
¼ cup chia or flax seeds
½ tablespoon ground cinnamon
¼ teaspoon salt
1 teaspoon vanilla extract
2 tablespoons canola or coconut oil
½ cup pure maple syrup
1 cup dried cranberries or other dried fruit (optional)

If possible, look for the dried ingredients at stores that sell in bulk.

Directions

1. Preheat oven to 325 F. Line a baking sheet with a silicone liner or parchment paper.
2. In a large bowl, combine all the dry ingredients. In a small bowl, stir together wet ingredients.
3. Pour wet ingredients over the dry ingredients and toss together until they are evenly coated.
4. Spread on lined baking sheet and bake for 30–45 minutes or until golden brown. Stir mixture every 10–15 minutes so the mixture cooks evenly.
5. Place baking sheet on a wire rack to cool. Granola will become crisp as it cools.

6. Once completely cooled, stir in dried fruit if desired. Store in an airtight container. It will keep in the refrigerator for several weeks. (We keep ours in a container outside the fridge and it gets eaten within days.)

* * *

Kell's Gazpacho
Recipe from Kell Killian

Ingredients

2 pounds tomatoes

1 peeled cucumber

½ green bell pepper

1 clove garlic

2 tablespoons sherry vinegar

1 teaspoon salt

2 tablespoons good quality olive oil

Directions

1. Blend all ingredients except olive oil.
2. Reblend with olive oil, adding more oil, vinegar or salt to taste.
3. Strain if desired (I never do).
4. Chill for at least one hour before serving.

References

Chapter 2

1. Hawken, P. (2017) *Drawdown: The Most Comprehensive Plan Ever Proposed to Reverse Global Warming* Penguin, 42.
2. ReFED, *2018 Annual Report*
3. Gerber, P.J., Steinfeld, H., Henderson, B., Mottet, A., Opio, C., Dijkman, J., Falcucci, A. & Tempio, G. (2013) *Tackling climate change through livestock – A global assessment of emissions and mitigation opportunities* Food and Agriculture Organization of the United Nations (FAO), Rome, 15.
4. U.S. Environmental Protection Agency, epa.gov/lmop/basic-information-about-landfill-gas.
5. U.S. Environmental Protection Agency, epa.gov/ghgemissions/understanding-global-warming-potentials.
6. Hawken, P., (2017) *Drawdown: The Most Comprehensive Plan Ever Proposed to Reverse Global Warming* Penguin, 39.
7. Mock, J. and Schwarz, J. (August 21, 2019) *What if We All Ate a Bit Less Meat* New York Times.
8. Bittman, M. (2009) *Food Matters: A Guide to Conscious Eating* Simon & Schuster Paperbacks; excerpt from on-line book description.
9. Hirsh, S. (July 26, 2019) *What is Heme? Impossible Foods' Magic Ingredient Has Caused Some Controversy* Green Matters.
10. Black, J. (Fall 2018) *Preventing Food Waste: What We Lose When Food Goes to Waste* World Wildlife Fund Magazine.
11. Ibid.

Chapter 3

1. Center for International Environmental Law (2019) *Plastic & Climate: The Hidden Costs of a Plastic Planet,* 3 and 19; ciel.org/plasticandclimate.
2. Snowden, S. (May 30, 2019) *300-Mile Swim Through the Great*

    Pacific Garbage Patch Will Collect Data on Plastic Pollution Forbes.

3. Ellen MacArthur Foundation (2017) *The New Plastics Economy: Rethinking the Future of Plastics.*

4. Abbing, M. R. (2019) *Plastic Soup: An Atlas of Ocean Pollution* Island Press.

5. The Climate Reality Project (October 23, 2018) *Ethane Cracker Plants: What Are They;* from blog: climaterealityproject.org/blog/ethane-cracker-plants-what-are-they.

6. United Nations Environment Programme (April 25, 2018) *From Birth to Ban: A History of the Plastic Shopping Bag* From website: unenvironment.org/news-and-stories.

7. Laville, S. (June 22, 2020) *Reusable Containers Safe During COVID-19 Pandemic, Say Experts* The Guardian.

Chapter 4

1. Katz, S. (March 2019) *Piling Up: How China's Ban on Importing Waste Has Stalled Global Recycling* Yale Environment 360.

2. Porter, B. (2018) *Reduce, Reuse, Reimagine: Sorting out the Recycling System* Rowman & Littlefield.

3. Paben, J. (November 21, 2019) *EPA: US recycled less plastic in 2017* Plastics Recycling Update.

4. Humes, E. (June 26, 2019) *The U.S. Recycling System is Garbage* Sierra Club Magazine.

5. Hocevar, J. (February 18, 2020) *Circular Claims Fall Flat: Comprehensive U.S. Survey of Plastics Recyclability* Greenpeace Reports

6. Based on my conversation with Beth Porter, author of (2018) *Reduce, Reuse, Reimagine: Sorting out the Recycling System* Rowman & Littlefield.

7. Hawken, P. (2017) *Drawdown: The Most Comprehensive Plan Ever Proposed to Reverse Global Warming* Penguin, 159.

8. U.S. Environmental Protection Agency (March 30, 2016) Environmental Factoids, WasteWise, archive.epa.gov/

epawaste/conserve/smm/wastewise/web/html/factoid.html

9. Porter, B. (2018) *Reduce, Reuse, Reimagine: Sorting out the Recycling System* Rowman & Littlefield, 88.

10. U.S. Environmental Protection Agency (March 30, 2016) Environmental Factoids, WasteWise, archive.epa.gov/wastes/conserve/tools/localgov/web/html/index-2.html.

11. Earth911 (September 3, 2015) *Earth911TV: Compostable Vs. Biodegradable Vs. Recyclable.*

Chapter 5

1. U.S. Environmental Protection Agency, epa.gov/facts-and-figures-about-materials-waste-and-recycling/textiles-material-specific-data.

2. McFall-Johnsen, M. (January 31, 2020) *These facts show how unsustainable the fashion industry is* World Economic Forum.

3. Goldstein, N. (August 23, 2008) *Changing Minds and Changing Towels* Psychology Today

4. World Meteorological Organization (March 11, 2020) *State of the Climate report released by the UN and WMO chiefs* public. wmo.int/en/media/news/state-of-climate-report-released-un-and-wmo-chiefs

References and Further Reading

Johnson, B. (2013) *A Zero Waste Home* Scribner

Hawken, P. (2017) Dra*wdown: The Most Comprehensive Plan Ever Proposed to Reverse Global Warming* Penguin

Project Drawdown, drawdown.org

Pollan, M. (2006) *The Omnivore's Dilemma* Penguin Books

Foer, J. (2019) *We are the Weather: Saving the Planet Begins at Breakfast* Farrar, Straus and Giroux

Kimball, C. (2018) *Milk Street Tuesday Nights* Little Brown and Company

Ottolenghi, Y. (2010) *Plenty* Chronicle Books

Ottolenghi, Y. (2014) *Plenty More* Ten Speed Press

Bittman, M. (2009) *Food Matters: A Guide to Conscious Eating* Simon & Schuster Paperbacks

Anne-Marie Bonneau, The Zero Waste Chef, zerowastechef.com

Compost Now, compostnow.org

Litterless litterless.com

The Institute for Local Self-Reliance ilsr.org/composting/map/

Porter, B. (2018) *Reduce, Reuse, Reimagine: Sorting out the Recycling System* Rowman & Littlefield

Kellogg, K. (2019) *101 Ways to Go Zero Waste* The Countryman Press

Bowman, T. (2020) *What if Solving the Climate Crisis is Simple?* Changemakers Books

Earth911 earth911.com

Miller, A. and Zaelke, D. (2020) *Cut Super Climate Pollutants Now!* Changemakers Books

About the Author

Stephanie Miller founded Zero Waste in DC to focus on the application of zero waste strategies that have a real and sustainable impact. With a goal of reaching as wide an audience as possible, she provides advisory services to individual households as well as community and corporate presentations. Within her 25-year career at the International Finance Corporation, the private sector arm of the World Bank Group, she served as Director of IFC's Climate Business Department where she led global teams to find innovative solutions to climate change.

Contact:
zerowasteindc.com
Instagram, Facebook, and Twitter: @zerowasteindc
linkedin.com/in/stephanie-j-miller

CHANGEMAKERS
BOOKS

TRANSFORMATION

Transform your life, transform your world – Changemakers
Books publishes for individuals committed to transforming
their lives and transforming the world. Our readers seek to
become
positive, powerful agents of change. Changemakers Books
inform, inspire, and provide practical wisdom and skills to
empower us to write the next chapter of humanity's future.
www.changemakers-books.com

The *Resilience* Series

The Resilience Series is a collaborative effort by the authors of Changemakers Books in response to the 2020 coronavirus epidemic. Each concise volume offers expert advice and practical exercises for mastering specific skills and abilities. Our intention is that by strengthening your resilience, you can better survive and even thrive in a time of crisis.
www.resilience-books.com

Adapt and Plan for the New Abnormal – in the COVID-19 Coronavirus Pandemic
Gleb Tsipursky

Aging with Vision, Hope and Courage in a Time of Crisis
John C. Robinson

Connecting with Nature in a Time of Crisis
Melanie Choukas-Bradley

Going Within in a Time of Crisis
P. T. Mistlberger

Grow Stronger in a Time of Crisis
Linda Ferguson

Handling Anxiety in a Time of Crisis
George Hoffman

Navigating Loss in a Time of Crisis
Jules De Vitto

The Life-Saving Skill of Story
Michelle Auerbach

Virtual Teams – Holding the Center When You Can't Meet Face-to-Face
Carlos Valdes-Dapena

Virtually Speaking – Communicating at a Distance
Tim Ward and Teresa Erickson

Current Bestsellers from Changemakers Books

Pro Truth
A Practical Plan for Putting Truth Back into Politics
Gleb Tsipursky and Tim Ward

How can we turn back the tide of post-truth politics, fake news, and misinformation that is damaging our democracy? In the lead up to the 2020 US Presidential Election, Pro Truth provides the answers.

An Antidote to Violence
Evaluating the Evidence
Barry Spivack and Patricia Anne Saunders

It's widely accepted that Transcendental Meditation can create peace for the individual, but can it create peace in society as a whole? And if it can, what could possibly be the mechanism?

Finding Solace at Theodore Roosevelt Island
Melanie Choukas-Bradley

A woman seeks solace on an urban island paradise in Washington D.C. through 2016-17, and the shock of the Trump election.

the bottom
a theopoetic of the streets
Charles Lattimore Howard

An exploration of homelessness fusing theology, jazz-verse and intimate storytelling into a challenging, raw and beautiful tale.

The Soul of Activism
A Spirituality for Social Change
Shmuly Yanklowitz

A unique examination of the power of interfaith spirituality to fuel the fires of progressive activism.

Future Consciousness
The Path to Purposeful Evolution
Thomas Lombardo

An empowering evolutionary vision of wisdom and the human mind to guide us in creating a positive future.

Preparing for a World that Doesn't Exist - Yet
Rick Smyre and Neil Richardson

This book is about an emerging Second Enlightenment and the capacities you will need to achieve success in this new, fast-evolving world.